DASH Diet

The Ultimate Guide to Everything DASH!

Jane Peters

The contents of this book may not be reproduced, duplicated or transmitted without direct written permission from the author.

Under no circumstances will any legal responsibility or blame be held against the publisher for any reparation, damages, or monetary loss due to the information herein, either directly or indirectly.

Legal Notice:

This book is copyright protected. This is only for personal use. You cannot amend, distribute, sell, use, quote or paraphrase any part or the content within this book without the consent of the author.

Disclaimer Notice:

Please note the information contained within this document is for educational and entertainment purposes only. Every attempt has been made to provide accurate, up to date and reliable complete information. No warranties of any kind are expressed or implied. Readers acknowledge that the author is not engaging in the rendering of legal, financial, medical or professional advice. The content of this book has been derived from various sources. Please consult a licensed professional before attempting any techniques outlined in this book.

By reading this document, the reader agrees that under no circumstances are is the author responsible for any losses, direct or indirect, which are incurred as a result of the use of information contained within this document, including, but not limited to, —errors, omissions, or inaccuracies.

Table of Contents

Chapter One

In-Depth Information About The Dash Diet

Introduction

There are numerous diet plans that have been proven to have important nutritional value to the human species in the contemporary world. On that note, nutritionists are striving to ensure that modern society is living a healthy life by educating them on diet matters. The need for people to improve their eating habits and live healthy has been on the rise. Perhaps it is for this reason that dietary knowledge has evolved to simpler menus and meals that can be utilized at home and at the restaurants. The content of this book expounds more on the DASH diet as one of the most prevalent, successful, and nutritious diets.

What is the DASH Diet?

Dietary Approaches to Stop Hypertension is abbreviated as DASH. The DASH diet plan is a strategy that entails eating low-fat meals. Additionally, the plan is designed to include a diet rich in fruits, vegetables, whole grains, and lean meats such as fish and poultry. Moreover, legumes and a limit on sugar-sweetened foods and beverages are also considered to be a vital ingredient of the diet plan. The DASH diet is a high fiber and low-fat plan.

The diet has been likened to the nutrition guidelines from the American-based National Heart, Lung, and Blood Institute which is part of the National Institutes of Health. The guidelines recommend meals with low sodium content along with vitamins and minerals. Although the benefits of the DASH diet are discussed further at a later part of this book, it is prudent to highlight that the plan is very effective in lowering blood pressure and cholesterol. Reduction of cholesterol in the body as a result of utilizing this plan goes a long way toward enhancing weight loss.

The DASH diet is a healthy way of eating patterns designed to be flexible and meet the lifestyle and food preferences of the larger part of the world's population. In many cases, dietary specialists and Registered Dietitian Nutritionists (RDNs) consider the DASH diet a version of the Mediterranean diet. However, the DASH diet has been made easier by more specific guidelines and precise recipes that can be followed to maximize the effects of the plan. There are more extensive versions of the DASH diet available that are mostly a result of personal discretion that can lower calories at a higher rate.

The History and Evolution of the DASH Diet

The history of the DASH diet plan dates back to 1992. The rise of hypertension in the American and world populace led doctors and nutritionists of that time to strive to look for solutions. In line with these efforts, the National Institutes of Health, based in the US, proposed a funding program to further research. The main research was to establish the role of dietary patterns on blood pressure.

The DASH diet research study used a meticulous design dubbed a randomized controlled trial (RCT). It was comprised of teams of the best physicians, nurses, nutritionists, statisticians, and research coordinators. The various teams were tasked to conduct research and come up with independent and viable dietary solutions to the hypertension problem. The research was conducted by five renowned medical research centers in different major cities in the US. These were:

- Johns Hopkins University in Baltimore,

Maryland

- Duke University Medical Center in Durham, North Carolina

- Kaiser Permanente Center for Health Research in Portland, Oregon

- Brigham and Women's Hospital in Boston, Massachusetts

- Pennington Biomedical Research Center in Baton Rouge, Louisiana

It is important to note that the researchers used two DASH trials: a standardized multi-center and a randomized outpatient feeding approach. Obviously, the main purpose of these two approaches was aligned to the main agenda to test the effect of dietary patterns on blood pressure.

The research was successfully completed in 1997 and that marked the beginning of the utilization of the DASH diet in the management of hypertension. The nutritional conceptualization of the DASH diet plan was based on this research. Further contemporary and advanced research has been carried out to establish other nutritional and medical benefits of this diet.

How to Get Started Implementing the DASH Diet into Your Life

The DASH diet works efficiently when you merge both your zeal to reap the benefits as well as commitment to procedures (recipes) as highlighted in this plan. The following are simple ways to get you started on the right track with the DASH diet:

- Ensure you consume more vegetables and fruits

- Regularly substitute refined grains for whole grains

- Frequently select fat-free or low-fat dairy products

- Make sure you choose lean protein sources like fish, poultry, and beans

- Try and consistently cook using vegetable oils

- Reduce your intake of foods which have high levels of added sugars, like soda and candy

- Cutoff the intake of foods highly saturated with fats like fatty meats, full-fat dairy, and oils like coconut and palm oil

- When possible, always add fresh, whole foods and more organic foods

To fully implement the DASH diet, establish an eating schedule containing the variety of foods recommended by the plan. This schedule is like a menu which should help you achieve more benefits from the DASH diet.

It is that easy! Now you can comfortably go on and use the DASH diet plan with ease.

Chapter Two

The Benefits Of The Dash Diet

How the DASH diet Lowers Your Blood Pressure

Using simpler words, blood pressure can be described as the measure of the force that the blood flowing inside blood vessels exerts on their walls. There are two major types of blood pressure:

1. Systolic pressure, which is the pressure exerted on the blood vessels when the heart beats.

2. Diastolic pressure, which is deemed the pressure in the blood vessels between heartbeats as well as when the heart is at rest.

In adults, the normal pressure levels for systolic pressure should be below 120 mmHg. Additionally, levels of diastolic pressure should be below 80 mmHg. Doctors always denote the overall blood pressure as a ratio of systolic blood pressure to diastolic pressure.

In order to help fight high levels of blood pressure, nutritionists prescribe the DASH diet plan to the patients. The diet has shown a clear indication of lowering blood pressure in both healthy people and those who already have high blood pressure. The DASH diet plan emphasizes maximizing the intake of foods that are rich in potassium, calcium, and magnesium. These minerals are vital to reducing blood pressure. Furthermore, the diet also discourages the consumption of salts and sodium minerals, thus reducing high levels of blood pressure. Although sodium is needed for many functions of the body, a large amount in the body may be lethal. The unutilized sodium minerals can cause fluid buildup which in turn strains the heart to efficiently pump blood. This situation makes blood pressure levels even worse.

Due to the fact that sodium consumption is not recommended, this contributes to lowering blood pressure even further. The reduction of salt intake as directed by the DASH diet plan has had an immense improvement in the reduction of blood pressure up to more than 10 points. Moreover, in people with normal blood pressure, the diet has reduced it by more than three points.

Although the diet can perfectly work to reduce blood pressure, it should not be mistaken for medication for the disorder. Always remember that high blood pressure kills! It is always prudent to consult with your doctor. Perhaps, after getting some medication to curb the high blood pressure, you can use the diet for a quick healing process.

Can You Lose Weight on the DASH Diet?

Even as many people are of the opinion that the DASH diet is not specially crafted for this, it is prudent to acknowledge the efforts of the diet on weight loss. If you already have been diagnosed with high blood pressure, chances are that your doctor has certainly advised you to burn more calories and lose weight. This is because the more your body weight, the higher your blood pressure is likely to be. In addition, shedding some weight has been proven to lower blood pressure. So, how can you lose weight using the DASH diet?

By lowering cholesterol

The inclusion of whole grains in the DASH diet presents the body with fiber content. An adequate level of fiber in the body reduces levels of cholesterol. Interestingly, high-fat dairy products work in the same way as fiber. The products shrink the level of triglycerides and cholesterol levels that can instigate diseases. Examples of foods with high levels of fiber include brown rice, wheat products, and oats.

By reducing calorie intake

In reference to the DASH diet plan, weight loss comes as a result of a caloric deficit. The diet is nutrient-dense oriented as opposed to calorie-rich meals thus helping in shedding off some pounds. Additionally, the DASH diet is a well-balanced diet filled with moderate levels of various nutrients and this is vital for the optimization of weight loss. Lowering the intake of processed fats and sweets and rising amounts of fruits, veggies, and low-fat dairy products can ultimately give the body abundant nutrients without feeling deprived or hungry. In turn, you are not going to eat within short intervals of time since the nutrients will make your stomach feel full. You still need to make sure you are eating fewer calories than you're burning.

How to Lose Weight on the DASH Eating Plan

The diet has been partially designed to help in losing weight. It is comprised of low-calorie foods such as fruits and vegetables. You can immensely lower caloric levels by replacing high-calorie foods with fruits and vegetables.

The following are general tips on how to lose weight while on the DASH diet.

1. Increase intake of fruits
    - It is better to eat a medium apple instead of several shortbread cookies
    - Snack on fruits, fresh vegetable sticks, unbuttered bread, and unsalted popcorn or sticks.
2. Increase vegetables in your meals
    - You can have a hamburger with carrots and some spinach leaves. When planning to eat chicken, add some raw vegetables and use a small amount of vegetable oil for frying.
3. When buying foods at the store, always use food labels to compare the fat content in packaged foods. It is prudent to note that items marked as low-fat or fat-free are not always lower in calories than their regular versions. Be on the lookout!
4. Reduce consumption of foods with high amounts of added sugar, such as regular soft drinks, pies, ice cream, flavored yogurts, and fruit drinks. Additionally, eat fruits canned in their own juice.

5. Use low-fat or fat-free condiments, such as fat-free salad dressings. You can also use pepper in small amounts during meals.

6. Select low-fat or fat-free dairy products to lower total fat intake.

    - Increase low-fat or fat-free dairy products. You can replace milk chocolate bars with low-fat frozen yogurt. This can help a lot in saving your body 100 calories per meal.

7. Eat smaller portions of foods during any meal. It is important to gradually cut back the volume of food eaten per meal rather than eating to fill your stomach as if there would be a food rationing afterward.

What are the Other Medical Benefits of the DASH Diet?

Over the years, the users of the DASH diet have attested to the various nutritional values it brings to the human body. Scientifically, the DASH diet is verified to be a very resourceful way to end numerous disorders that cause health complications. However, there are no reports put forth by any users that link the DASH diet to negative effects. The following are the major benefits that curb rampant killer diseases.

Enhanced heart health

High blood pressure is dangerous due to the fact that it has an immense impact on the heart and how it works. High blood pressure increases chances of strokes and heart attacks. This can be attributed to the excess strain on blood vessels and arteries of the cardiovascular system by blood as it flows under high pressure. The DASH diet plan reduces all these risks by encouraging intake of more fiber and low-cholesterol foods.

Inhibits osteoporosis

Osteoporosis is a medical condition that makes bone fragile. The condition increases chances of bones being susceptible to fractures. The DASH diet is comprised of a high calcium, protein, and potassium content. These minerals are essential in preventing or curtailing the onset of osteoporosis. To aid in making bones stronger, the diet recommends the intake of milk, lean proteins, grains, leafy vegetables, and fruits. All these foods contribute sufficient levels of the mentioned minerals. If you want to develop strong bones and at the same time reap all these other benefits, then subscribing to the DASH diet is a superb idea.

Increasing kidney health

Over the recent past, the DASH diet has been linked to

the prevention and reduction of kidney stones. People who experience kidney stones can attest that they are very painful and can lead to malfunctioning kidneys. The diet is designed to lessen the intake of sodium which is known to cause kidney stones. Basically, doctors have explained that sodium dehydrates the body and overworks the kidneys, leading to kidney stones. If the DASH diet does not work positively to end the kidney stones, the patient should visit a specialist for advanced treatment.

Prevents cancer

Another benefit of the DASH diet is its indisputable impact on certain cancers. The high content of whole grains, fruits, and vegetables translates to a high concentration of fiber, vitamins, and antioxidants. These nutrients can prevent the impact of the byproducts of cellular respiration that causes mutation in healthy cells and lead to the spread of cancer.

Diabetes Care

The revised version of the DASH diet suggests an efficient way of eliminating the empty carbohydrates and starchy foods from your meals. One way is by avoiding high levels of simple sugars that the body can easily absorb and remit to the bloodstream. This is what regulates the glucose and insulin levels in the body thus reducing any chances of getting diabetes. According to a number of nutritionists and doctors, diabetes is a precursor of everything from obesity and cancer to heart disease. Due to this, diabetes is to be fought at all cost.

Prevention of depression

Advanced research which has always been done to make the diet better has noted that it reduces the chances of getting depression. Facts from various researchers have shown that consumption of a diet comprising fruits, vegetables, and whole grains enhances proper brain function as well as enhancing how depression is dealt with. Even as you are mesmerized by the listed benefits of the DASH diet, the chronic conditions mentioned above need the attention of a doctor. The ideal thing to do is to boost the medication given by the doctor with the diet rather than use the diet as a medication. Nutrition is a key aspect of all health concerns, but changing your diet can be disastrous unless applied cautiously. Therefore, it is crucial to seek advice from your medical professional or a nutritionist before making any drastic changes to your diet.

Chapter Three

Eating Out Versus Cooking In Your Kitchen

Tips for Eating Out

Once in a blue moon, it is blissful to go out and enjoy a meal in a restaurant or a food joint that satisfies your stomach with a variety of delicacies on their menu. However, it does not mean that you should forget that you are on the DASH diet and overindulge. You may think that it is only for one meal or one day but the damage made will be retrogressive to the benefits of the diet. Perhaps it may take a few weeks to recuperate. The following are tips for eating while on an outing.

Restrain Yourself from Salty Foods

A primary recommendation of the DASH diet is to cut the consumption of salt. Salt is rampantly used to enhance flavor in meals. Therefore, the use of salt in a restaurant is not an exception. When you go out for lunch or dinner, make sure that you order foods that are less likely to have salt. Moreover, when you get food with a lower salt level that you expected, hold yourself back from using the salt shaker. Again, limit the amounts of condiments that are rich in salts like ketchup, sauces, and mustard. Ask for lemon and fresh herbs for seasonings.

Do Not Order High-Fat Content Foods

Preferably, order foods that are low in saturated fat and which don't have high levels of calories. To be more precise, ask whether the restaurant has food fried with olive oil rather than corn oil. Moreover, if you intend to eat a burger or any other snack, skip the cheese or butter that may be an ingredient. When eating meat, trim off visible fat parts. You can also request steamed, rather than deep-fried, fish.

Avoid Overeating

The DASH diet is designed to limit the portions of food consumed in a meal. On the other hand, restaurants are fond of serving us with their standard amounts. In most instances, these amounts are more than we can consume.

When on the DASH diet and eating out, share the extra portion with a friend. If alone, put a share of the meal in a takeout container before eating.

Exert Caution While Eating Fast Foods

Even as you are on the DASH diet, you can occasionally enjoy fast foods. Conversely, the amounts of these foods should be consumed in moderation. Ensure that you do not add salt to these foods. You could use some lemons for seasoning. It would be reckless for you to order a meal with unhealthy extras, such as cheese or butter dressing.

NOTE: These are only a few tips. Use your discretion to ensure you reduce the intake of those foods and items that are not recommended by the DASH diet.

Cooking In Your Kitchen

When you find it difficult to go out, for whatever reason, you can always prepare a delicious meal in your kitchen. This topic expounds more on the grocery buying list, the 30-day meal plan, and the recipes that you can follow to teach you to make finger-licking delicacies in your kitchen.

1. **The Grocery list; Foods you can eat while**

on the DASH diet

People who have not tried the DASH diet are of the notion that the recommended ingredients are expensive and rare to find in the market. This is a wrong notion since these ingredients are even readily available in the grocery store near you. These items are not costly and can be purchased while sticking to a low budget.

The following are some items that are highly suggested by the DASH diet. They have proven to be very efficient in giving and maintaining nutritional values as required by the DASH diet.

1. **Vegetables**
   They are very rich in magnesium, potassium, healthy vitamins, and fiber.

   Examples are:

   - Broccoli
   - Carrots
   - Squash
   - Tomatoes
   - Sweet potatoes
   - Brussels
   - Sprouts
   - Spinach
   - Cucumbers
   - Kale

- Green beans

Buying tip: always ensure that levels of sodium and salt on canned or frozen veggies are thoroughly checked.

2. **Fruits**

   Fruits are a great source of fiber, potassium, and magnesium minerals.

   Examples are:
   - Bananas
   - Apples
   - Grapes
   - Berries
   - Oranges
   - Pineapples

Buying tip: always confirm that canned fruits have no added flavors or synthetic added sugars.

3. **Fat-free Dairy products**

   Dairy produce provides abundant sources of proteins, calcium, and vitamin D.

   Examples are:
   - Fresh milk
   - Cream
   - Yogurt
   - Cheese

Buying tip: always check that you are buying a low-fat dairy product for the DASH diet plan.

4. **Nuts, seeds, and legumes**

    These items are sources of high levels of protein, magnesium, and potassium minerals. The photochemical plant compounds contained by these items are said to be helpful in protecting and taming certain types of cancer and cardiovascular diseases.

    Examples are:
    - Peas
    - Black beans
    - Lentils
    - Sunflower seeds
    - Almonds
    - Kidney beans
    - Walnuts
    - Pistachios

Buying tip: at all times, avoid high-fat content seeds or nuts like coconuts.

5. **Fats and Oils**

    Fats help the body in enhancing the absorption of vitamins.

    Examples are:
    - Olive oil

- Margarine
- Canola oil
- Low-fat mayonnaise
- Safflower oil

Buying tip: check to ensure that margarine and salad dressing have the lowest levels of fat.

6. **Grains**

    They are known for their richness in fiber content. Examples are:

    - Quinoa
    - Pasta
    - Brad
    - Cereal
    - Brown rice
    - Whole grain cereal

Buying tip: avoid processed grains which might have butter, cream, or cheese spreads.

It is wise to note that all these ingredients are bought at a person's discretion. By this, we mean that the quantities and volumes to be bought should be perhaps based on the money you have or the space in your fridge.

Any person using this book as a guideline for achieving the best from the DASH diet should note that the items listed above are just a few examples. More items under each category can be obtained from the market. In a later chapter, recipes are included to help you make the listed ingredients into a superb meal for breakfast, lunch, or dinner.

The following are tips to suggest an effective way of utilizing the DASH diet without depleting your bank account.

1. Have a plan for every meal and make a list of all the ingredients you need to buy. This will help keep you from impulse buying.
2. Always have a preference for unprocessed food in place of processed foods. This is because processed foods are more expensive and may contain unhealthy components.
3. Most grocery stores give promotional discounts that you may take advantage of and purchase in bulk. You can buy more items that can take you up to the next big promotion. However, do not be excited about these offers and forget that large quantities of groceries may not fit in your home freezer.
4. Planta home garden where you can grow your own vegetables. You can also develop a yard for some fruit plants. This can help in saving you some money which could be used in buying the items from a store.

5. Avoid convenience foods like pre-cut fruits and vegetables. If you do a critical cost analysis of buying these sliced foods, you will notice that they are costlier as compared to buying the whole item.

6. Buy from the local farmers in your neighborhood. They are the best in giving you farm-fresh produce at a very low and affordable cost.

7. Make a habit of cooking at home instead of eating out. It is evident that eating out can be more expensive than cooking at home. It doesn't mean that you are stingy! It only translates to cost-saving. Actually, you might be fascinated that the cost of one meal at a restaurant can buy ingredients for around three meals for the DASH diet plan.

8. In the cooking schedule, skip meat on specified days. Buying meat every day and for every meal can drain your bank account so fast that you will not even notice it. Replace meat with other ingredients that are rich in protein like beans, peas, and lentils.

30-Day Meal DASH Diet Plan

The following schedule can be used to ensure that you keep up the use of DASH diet meals within the month.

Basically, the plan plays the role of a menu which should be employed while determining the needed ingredients and making meals. This 30-day DASH diet plan can be repeated for around three consecutive months for better results.

	Breakfast	Lunch	Dinner
Day 1	Banana pecan compote	Rice noodles with spring vegetables	Quick bean and tuna salad
Day 2	Cranberry orange glaze	Veggie pizza	Chicken adobo soup with bok choy
Day 3	Almond and apricot biscotti	Smoky bean and mushroom cornucopias	Roasted turkey with balsamic sauce
Day 4	Apple lettuce salad	Vegetarian kebabs	Beef and vegetable kebabs
Day 5	Grilled mango chutney	Turkey bean soup	Brown rice pilaf
Day 6	Buckwheat pancakes	Tomato basil pesto sauce	Curried carrot soup
Day 7	Best honey whole-wheat bread	Vegetable lasagna roll-ups	Fried rice
Day 8	Spiced carrot raisin bread	Hot ham and cheese sandwiches with mushrooms	Grilled chicken salad with olives and oranges

Day 9	Three-grain raspberry muffins	Rice and beans salad	Green beans with red pepper and garlic
Day 10	Ham, pineapple, and asparagus crepes	Hearty turkey chili	Chicken Caesar pitas
Day 11	Whole-wheat blueberry pancakes	Pita pizza	Broccoli with garlic and lemon
Day 12	Veggie egg bake	Turkey and broccoli crepe	Brussels sprouts with shallots and lemon
Day 13	Overnight refrigerator oatmeal	Marinated Portobello mushrooms with provolone	Braised celery root
Day 14	Spinach and mushroom frittata	Steak with chimichurri sauce	Paella with chicken, leeks, and tarragon
Day 15	Sweet potato soufflé	Grilled turkey burger	Turkey breast burgers
Day 16	Buckwheat pancakes	Tomato basil pesto sauce	Curried carrot soup
Day 17	Best honey whole-wheat bread	Vegetable lasagna roll-ups	Fried rice
Day 18	Spiced carrot raisin bread	Hot ham and cheese sandwiches with mushrooms	Grilled chicken salad with olives and oranges

Day 19	Three-grain raspberry muffins	Rice and beans salad	Green beans with red pepper and garlic
Day 20	Banana pecan compote	Rice noodles with spring vegetables	Quick bean and tuna salad
Day 21	Cranberry orange glaze	Veggie pizza	Chicken adobo soup with bok choy
Day 22	Almond and apricot biscotti	Smoky bean and mushroom cornucopias	Roasted turkey with balsamic sauce
Day 23	Best honey whole-wheat bread	Vegetable lasagna roll-ups	Fried rice
Day 24	Spiced carrot raisin bread	Hot ham and cheese sandwiches with mushrooms	Grilled chicken salad with olives and oranges
Day 25	Three-grain raspberry muffins	Rice and beans salad	Green beans with red pepper and garlic
Day 26	Ham, pineapple, and asparagus crepes	Hearty turkey chili	Chicken Caesar pitas
Day 27	Spinach and mushroom frittata	Steak with chimichurri sauce	Paella with chicken, leeks, and tarragon

Day 28	Sweet potato soufflé	Grilled turkey burger	Turkey breast burgers
Day 29	Buckwheat pancakes	Tomato basil pesto sauce	Curried carrot soup
Day 30	Best honey whole-wheat bread	Vegetable lasagna roll-ups	Fried rice

***The plan can be repeated within the 30 days. Moreover, any other foods that are found on other sources of the DASH Diet nutrition information can be added to this plan.**

Chapter Four

Weight Loss

Indicators that You Need to Lose Weight

You may be wondering what specifically determines if you need to lose some weight. The following are some pointers that will help you conclude that truly, you have gained unnecessary weight that you may need to shed.

1. **Advice from the doctor or nutritionist**
    You may be feeling as if you are not sure whether you need to lose some weight or not. The ideal thing to do is to confirm with your doctor or nutritionist. This way, you shall get a sure answer that will tell you how much you have gained, how much you need to lose, and any viable means to lose it.

2. **When you snore while sleeping**
    Doctors and nutritionist have established that snoring while sleeping is sometimes a result of obstructive sleep apnea which usually results

from excess weight or obesity. If you are snoring while sleeping, this is the time that you start working on a plan to lose some weight. However, there is another condition that blocks your sinuses and may cause snoring. This is a medical condition and should get the attention of a specialist.

3. **When you find it hard to exercise**
    Becoming heavy as a result of weight gain can make exercising turn out to be a challenging affair. In addition, your self-conscious will tell you not to go the gym because you can feel the extra weight since you do not like to be seen out of shape. This is a clear indication that you have added weight that needs to be lost.

4. **After finding out you have added several pounds**
    It's always convenient when walking on the street and you meet a person with a scale which only requires a few coins. When you weigh yourself and notice that you have added some more weight, it is time to make necessary changes to your diet and exercising patterns.

5. **When your body mass index indicates elevated numbers**
    The body mass index (BMI) is the measure of your body fat based on the height and weight.

When it increases, it basically means that you have gained weight. This should automatically become a clear indication that you need to lose weight within the next few weeks to get back to normal.

6. **When your clothes do not fit you anymore**
   When you cannot fit into those jeans that you bought when you were in shape, it means your body has gained some weight. It is inevitable to lose weight if at all you want your initial body weight back.

7. **When you develop aching joints**
   Increased body fat exerts more pressure on your bones and joints and can wear down tissues around them. As a result, the pressure is felt as pain. Working out not only enables you to lose weight but will also enhance the movement of your joints.

Importance of Exercising

Sometimes, we fail to clearly comprehend the importance of exercising or why we even have to exercise. Working out is an important thing not only to lose weight and get a desired shape and size but also to have a healthy impact on the human body. Below are benefits of exercising that should remind us why we need a schedule and to regularly avail ourselves of workouts.

Controlling weight

Since time immemorial, exercising is the commonest way been used for shedding some unnecessary added weight. Exercise enhances excess weight loss and maintains a desired body shape and size. According to science, the more you workout, the more calories you lose. Exercising does not necessarily mean that you have to visit a gym. Surprisingly, you can use the stairs at your home to work out. Going up and down the stairs several times is enough exercise for a day. Moreover, taking up more household chores can also help you work out your muscles.

Increases energy levels

Exercise boosts both the strength and the efficiency of the cardiovascular system. This makes the flow of oxygen and nutrients to your muscles better. According to doctors, when the cardiovascular system is in good working condition, everything becomes easier and your body generates more energy. In addition, exercising boosts your endurance which can really help you have more energy to tackle daily chores.

Exercise tackles health conditions and diseases

Working out is a good way to manage a series of health problems that have become rampant in the modern world. Some diseases that can be reduced using exercise are metabolic syndrome, stroke, type 2 diabetes, depression, arthritis, and a number of different types of cancers. Even as exercising helps to lessen the propagation of these diseases in your body, it should not be mistaken for a kind of medication. It would be wise to get a checkup in order to get the best medical care from your doctor.

Improved brain function

Exercising increases the efficiency of blood flow and oxygen levels in the human brain. It also has proven to be an exceedingly conducive way for enhancing the release of brain chemicals that are responsible for various body functions. For example, the enhancement of production of cells in the hippocampus, which is the brain part that controls memory. In turn, this increases concentration levels and cognitive abilities. Exercising is the most recommended way to fight the risk of cognitive degenerative diseases such as Alzheimer's.

Boosts the working condition of the heart

High blood pressure is a result of the heart straining to

pump blood through the blockage of the arteries which is mainly caused by high levels of cholesterol in the body. Exercising greatly reduces the pressure on your heart as well as maintaining the good form of the heart muscles. This is because of the drastic reduction of the LDL cholesterol that clogs the blood arteries. The development of coronary heart disease can be reduced when exercise is combined with healthy and cholesterol-free diets.

Rejuvenate your sex life

Engaging in sex is a more of a physical activity than it is a mental affair. This means that you need to have the morale and strength needed. In order to have the required body strength, you need to work out and restore your muscles. According to sex therapists, regular physical activity can be helpful in enhancing arousal for women. Moreover, it has also been noted that men who work out frequently are less likely to develop problems that are deemed as the origin of erectile dysfunction.

Enhances the immune system

As mentioned earlier, exercising reduces the logjam of blood arteries. This helps in improving the heart's ability to sufficiently pump oxygen and nutrients around the body. The more you workout, the more you consequently boost the required nutrients which fuel the growth of cells that fight bacteria and viruses from attacking the immune system.

Promotes better sleep

Even as many people follow the philosophy that sleeping will never get you rich, good sleeping patterns can make you healthier. Good quality sleep goes a long way toward improving the overall wellness of the brain by reducing stress. Regular physical activity helps you to fall asleep easier and deepens your sleep. This is because after exercising, your body is tired and ready to be put to rest.

Helps to prevent and treat mental illnesses

Mental illness can range from frustrations to depression, acute loss of memory, and concentration. We all have different ways to deal with stress, which easily leads to depression. However, the healthiest way is exercise. Actually, as most people workout, they do so to 'wrestle' their frustrations and what is on their mind. This, in turn, relieves the brain from any possible illness.

Exercise creates fun

Exercising and physical activity gives you a chance to let everything go, enjoy the outdoors, or simply engage in activities that make you ecstatic. Additionally, physical activity can help you link up with family members or friends in a fun social setting. Therefore, you should take a dance class, jog around the park, hit the hiking trails, or join a soccer team as a form of exercise. You will definitely get in high spirits and eliminate boredom.

It is advisable to workout with moderation. If you go to the gym for your workouts, refrain from lifting heavy weights that may tear your muscles. Aim to exercise for around 1 to 2 hours per day. This is enough time to ensure that you attain the desired impact. Moreover, it is good to combine both vigorous and moderate aerobic exercises such as walking, running, and swimming. Additionally, squeeze in strength training at least twice per week. This can be by lifting free weights, using weight machines, or doing body weight exercises.

Remember to consult with your nutritionist or doctor before commencing a new exercise program. This ensures your selection is safe for your health especially if you have chronic health problems or have not exercised for a long time.

Chapter Five

60 Dash Diet Recipes

15 Breakfast recipes

15 Lunch recipes

15 Dinner recipes

15 Snack recipes

15 Breakfast Recipes

Banana pecan compote

Number of Servings: 6

Ingredients

- 4 very ripe sliced medium bananas
- 2full tablespoons brown sugar
- 1/2a cup orange juice
- 1teaspoon vanilla
- 1/2a teaspoon cinnamon
- 2 tablespoons chopped pecans

Instructions

Heat a medium-sized saucepan to moderate heat

1. Add bananas and the brown sugar and stir-fry for about 1 to 2 minutes. Do this until all the sugar dissolves.
2. Add some orange juice, cinnamon, and vanilla.
3. Let the orange juice reduce for around two minutes
4. Sprinkle the pecans over the mixture prior to serving.

Nutritional Information per Serving

Serving Amount: 1/3 cup

Calories	109	Monounsaturated fat	1g
Protein	1 g	Cholesterol	0mg
Total fat	2 g	Sodium	2mg
Saturated fat	0g	Total carbohydrate	24g
Trans fat	0g	Dietary fiber	2g
Total sugars	14g		

Cranberry orange glaze

Number of Servings:4

Ingredients

- 1cup fresh cranberries, chopped
- 2/3 cup unsweetened orange juice
- 1 tablespoon cornstarch
- Sugar substitute

Instructions

1. Combine the orange juice, cornstarch, and cranberries in a microwave bowl.
2. Continue stirring until the mixture thickens.
3. Stir a number of times as you continue to cook the mixture in the microwave. After 4 to 5minutes, set aside to cool.
4. Add the sugar substitute and taste.
5. Ensure that the glaze is sour. Serve over chicken, pork, and turkey.
6. This combination can be used as a great sauce for grilling, a marinade, or for roasting.

Nutritional Information per Serving

Serving Amount: 1/4cup

Calories	36	Sodium	1mg
Cholesterol	10g	Total carbohydrate	9g
Saturated fat	0g	Dietary fiber	1g
Trans fat	0g	Monounsaturated fat	0g
Added sugars	0g	Total fat	0g

Grilled mango chutney

Number of Servings:6

Ingredients

- 1mango, peeled and pitted
- 1/4cup sugar
- 1/4cup chopped red onion
- 2tablespoons cider vinegar
- 2 tablespoons finely chopped green bell pepper
- 2tablespoon grated fresh ginger
- 1/2 teaspoon ground ginger
- 1/8 teaspoon ground cloves
- 1/4teaspoon chopped fresh rosemary

Instructions

1. Set up a hot fire in a charcoal grill.
2. Away from this heat source, gently coat the grill rack with cooking spray. Place the cooking rack 4 to 6 inches from the heat source.
3. Fix the mango on the grill rack and ensure only moderate heat is getting to it.
4. Turn often until the mango is browned on each side. This should be after around 3-4 minutes.
5. After this, remove the mango from the rack and allow it to cool for a few minutes.

6. Place the mango on a chopping board and cut it into smaller chunks. Put the pieces into a bowl.
7. Add the other ingredients into the bowl and stir to mix
8. Cover the bowl and refrigerate for about 1 hour. This will enhance absorption of sugar.
9. Serve as a relish for rice, meat, and poultry.
10. Cover and refrigerate until sugar is absorbed and flavors mingle, about 1 hour.
11. Serve as a relish for meat, poultry, or rice.

Nutritional Information per Serving

Serving Amount: 2 serving spoons

Calories	58	Trans fat	0g
Cholesterol	0mg	Carbohydrate	15g
Sodium	1mg	Added sugars	8g
Dietary fiber	1g		

Apple lettuce salad

Number of Servings:4

Ingredients

- 1/4cup unsweetened apple juice
- 2 tablespoons lemon juice
- 1 tablespoon canola oil
- Two 1/4 teaspoons brown sugar
- 1/2 teaspoon Dijon mustard
- 1/4 teaspoon apple pie spice
- 1 medium red apple chopped
- 8cups mixed salad greens

Instructions

1. Combine the apple juice, brown sugar, lemon juice, mustard, and apple pie spice in a salad bowl.
2. Sprinkle the canola oil on the mixture and stir to mix evenly
3. Add apple and flip to coat.
4. Add salad greens and flip again to mix before serving.

Nutritional Information per Serving

Serving Amount: 2 cups lettuce and 1/4 cup apple

Calories	115	Dietary fiber	3g
Sodium	44mg	Total fat	4g
Added sugars	5g	Saturated fat	0g
Monounsaturated fat	2g	Trans fat	0g
Cholesterol	0mg	Protein	1g
Total carbohydrate	19g		

Almond and apricot biscotti

Number of Servings: Two - Four

Ingredients

- 3/4 cup whole-meal flour
- 3/4cup all-purpose plain flour
- 1/4 cup firmly packed brown sugar
- 1 teaspoon baking powder
- 2 eggs, lightly beaten
- 2 tablespoons one percent low-fat milk
- 2 tablespoons canola oil
- 2 tablespoons dark honey
- 1/2 teaspoon almond extract
- 2/3 cup chopped dried apricots
- 1/4 coarsely chopped almonds

Instructions

1. Start by pre-heating the oven to 175 C.
2. Combine the brown sugar, baking powder, and the flours in a bowl. Fluff to blend
3. Add the canola oil, eggs, milk, honey and almond extract in any order. You should then stir with a wooden spoon until the dough starts to form.
4. To the dough, add the cut apricots and almonds. Using floured hands, mix the dough until it is well-blended.

5. Position the dough on a long sheet of plastic wrap. Using your hand, shape the dough into a flattened log measuring 12-inches long, 3-inches wide, and about 1-inch high.
6. Lift the plastic wrap to turn the dough upside down onto a nonstick baking sheet.
7. Bake for 25 to 30 minutes until it turns to lightly browned. Transfer the dough to another baking sheet to cool for around 10 minutes. Leave the oven set at the initial 175 C.
8. Place the cooled log on a cutting board and cut crosswise on the diagonal to make 24 pieces.
9. Arrange the slices on the baking sheet with the cut-side down. Return to the oven and bake for 15 to 20 minutes until the dough turns crispy.
10. Move to a wire rack and let cool completely and afterwards store in an airtight container.

Nutritional Information per Serving

Serving Amount: 1 cookie

Calories	75	Sodium	17mg
Monounsaturated fat	1g	Total carbohydrate	12g
Cholesterol	15mg	Total sugars	6g
Dietary fiber	1g	Added sugars	2g
Protein	2g		

Buckwheat pancakes

Number of Servings: 6

Ingredients

- 2egg whites
- 1tablespoon canola oil
- 1/2 cup fat-free milk
- 1/2 cup all-purpose plain flour
- 1/2 cup buckwheat flour
- 1 tablespoon baking powder
- 1 tablespoon sugar
- 1/2 cup sparkling water
- 3 cups sliced fresh strawberries

Instructions

1. Whisk the egg whites, canola oil, and milk together in a small bowl
2. Combine the sugar, flours, and baking powder in another bowl.
3. Add the sparkling water into the egg white mixture and stir.
4. Place a nonstick frying pan on a grill under medium heat.
5. Sprinkle 1/2 cup pancake batter into the pan when a drop of water hisses and hits the pan.

6. Cook for around 2-3 minutes until the edges are lightly browned and the surface of the pancake is covered with bubbles.
7. Cook and turn until the bottom is well-browned.
8. Repeat the same procedure with the remaining pancake batter.
9. Transfer the cooked pancakes to another plate.
10. Cover each pancake with 1/2 cup of sliced strawberries.
11. Serve immediately.

Nutritional Information per Serving

Serving Amount: 2 small pancakes

Calories	143	Total carbohydrate	24g
Total fat	3g	Sodium	150mg
Monounsaturated fat	2g	Dietary fiber	3g
Protein	5g	Total sugars	6.5g
Trans fat	0g	Added sugars	2g

Best honey whole-wheat bread

Number of Servings: at least 5 per loaf

Ingredients

- 1 cup dry rolled oats
- 3 cups water
- 3 cups whole-wheat flour
- 3/4 cup soy flour
- 3/4 cup ground flaxseed or flaxseed meal
- 3 tablespoons sesame seeds
- 3 tablespoons poppy seeds
- Four 1/4 tablespoons yeast
- 1 tablespoon sea salt
- 1 cup unsweetened applesauce
- 1/2 cup honey
- 1/4 cup olive oil
- About 5 cups unbleached white flour

Instructions

1. Put dry rolled oats mixed with water in a microwave-safe bowl and heat to about 50-60C.
2. Combine the ground flaxseed, whole-wheat flour, soy flour, sesame and poppy seeds, yeast, , and salt. Stir thoroughly to mix.

3. Add applesauce, honey, and oil and mix by hand. Afterwards, add the hot rolled oats mixture and continue mixing by hand.
4. When properly blended, use a dough hook mixer to stir for about 3 minutes.
5. Slowly, add (sprinkle) some white flour until dough detaches from sides of bowl and turn out to be smooth and elastic.
6. Cover dough in bowl and put it in a warm place.
7. For about one and a half to two hours, let the dough rise until about double in size. Hit the dough down and divide it into 4 pieces.
8. Shape the dough into 4 loaves and place into 2 ½ x 4½ x 8 ½-inch loaf pans sprayed with cooking spray. You could repeat one size of the loaf pans.
9. Cover the pans and place in a warm spot.
10. Bake at 175C for 25 minutes or until the covers of loaves turn golden.
11. Remove the loaves from the pans and cool on a rack. Cut into half-inch-wide slices and serve.

Nutritional Information per Serving

Serving Amount: ½ -inch slice

Calories	90	Cholesterol	0mg
Dietary fiber	2g	Sodium	104mg
Saturated fat	0.2g	Total fat	2g
Protein	3g	Trans fat	0g
Total carbohydrate	15g	Added sugars	2g
Monounsaturated fat	1g		

Spiced carrot raisin bread

Number of Servings: 8

Ingredients

- 1 1/2cup whole-wheat pastry flour
- 1/2 teaspoon baking soda
- 1 1/2teaspoons baking powder
- 1/2 teaspoon salt
- 1 tablespoon cinnamon
- 1/2 teaspoon nutmeg
- 1/4 teaspoon cloves
- 1/4teaspoon paprika or cayenne
- 1tablespoon grated lemon zest
- 1/4cup ground flaxseed
- 2eggs
- 1/2 cup brown sugar
- 1/4 cup honey
- 1/2 cup unsweetened applesauce
- 1/4cup olive oil
- 3/4 teaspoon almond extract
- 2 cups shredded carrots
- 2/3 cup raisins

Instructions

1. Preheat oven to 190 C.

2. Whisk the baking powder, salt, spices, flour and baking soda in a large bowl.

3. In a separate bowl, mix honey, lemon zest, applesauce, olive oil, eggs, sugar, and almond extract.

4. When all these ingredients have been mixed properly, add carrots, flaxseeds and raisins.

5. Mix the wet and dry ingredients until they have been perfectly combined while being careful not to overmix.

6. **Pour batter into a greased9 x 5-inch loaf pan and bake at 190 C for around 45 minutes to one hour.**

7. Cut into half an inch slices and serve.

Nutritional Information per Serving

Serving Amount: 1 half-inch thick slice

Calories	136	Total carbohydrate	22g
Sodium	150mg	Dietary fiber	2g
Saturated fat	0.5g	Trans fat	0g
Total fat	4g	Protein	3g
Cholesterol	21mg	Added sugars	8g
Monounsaturated fat	2.5g		

Three-grain raspberry muffins

Number of Servings:12

Ingredients

- 1/2 cup rolled oats
- 1 cup low-fat milk or plain soy milk
- 3/4cup all-purpose flour
- 1/2 cup cornmeal, preferably stone-ground
- 1/4cup wheat bran
- 1tablespoon baking powder
- 1/4 teaspoon salt
- 1/2 cup dark honey
- 3 ½ tablespoons canola oil
- 2 teaspoons grated lime zest
- 1egg, lightly beaten
- 2/3 cup raspberries

Instructions

1. Preheat the oven to 200C.
2. Grease a 12-cup muffin pan with some oil and line with foil.
3. Combine the oats and milk in a microwave-safe bowl of considerable size.
4. Cook in the microwave oven for around 3 minutes until the oats are creamy and tender and set aside.

5. In a separate bowl, combine the salt, cornmeal, baking powder, all-purpose flour and bran. Whisk the mixture to blend.

6. Add the canola oil, lime zest, honey, and oats mixture followed by an egg.

7. Beat the mixture until it dampens but is still a little lumpy. Now, gently fold in the raspberries.

8. Spoon out the batter into the muffin cups and make each cup about 2/3 full.

9. Bake for around 16 to 18 minutes or until the muffins develop a golden-brown color. You can check whether the muffins are well-cooked by using a toothpick inserted into the center of a muffin. If completely cooked, it will come out clean.

10. To ensure that the cooked muffins cool, transfer them to a wire rack for around 10-20 minutes.

Nutritional Information per Serving

Serving Amount: 1 muffin

Calories	165	Sodium	126mg
Cholesterol	16mg	Saturated fat	0.5g
Dietary fiber	2g	Monounsaturated fat	3g
Protein	3g	Added sugars	11g
Trans fat	Less than 0.5g	Total fat	5g
Total carbohydrate	27g		

Ham, pineapple, and asparagus crepes

Number of Servings:4

Ingredients

- 6 asparagus stalks, halved
- 4pre-packaged crepes, each about 8 inches in diameter
- 8 ounces reduced-sodium, extra-lean ham, thinly sliced
- 1/2 cup crushed pineapple, drained of juice
- 1/2 cup shredded reduced-fat cheese

Instructions

1. Put onto the oven and heat it to about 150C.
2. Sparingly, spread cooking spray on a baking dish
3. In a separate pot fitted with a steamer basket, boil some water and add asparagus. Cover and steam for about 2-3 minutes
4. Heat the crepes in a microwave for up to a maximum of 1 minute.
5. Place a small amount of ham, 2 full tablespoons pineapple, 2 tablespoons cheese, and 3 steamed asparagus stalks in each crepe.
6. In the prepared baking dish, roll up the crepes and place seam-side down.

7. Bake the ingredients for about 3-5 minutes until the cheese starts to melt.

8. Cool for around 5 minutes and serve

Nutritional Information per Serving

Serving Amount: 1 crepe

Calories	253	Saturated fat	6g
Cholesterol	127mg	Sodium	742mg
Total fat	13g	Monounsaturated fat	4g
Dietary fiber	1g	Total carbohydrate	21g
Added sugars	0g	Total sugars	9g
Protein	18g	Trans fat	0g

Whole-wheat blueberry pancakes

Number of Servings:6

Ingredients

- 1 ¾ cup white whole-wheat flour
- 2teaspoons baking powder
- 1tablespoon sugar
- 1/2 teaspoon cinnamon
- 1 ¾ cup skim milk
- 1 egg, lightly beaten
- 1tablespoon canola oil
- 1 cup fresh or frozen whole blueberries

Instructions

1. Combine cinnamon, sugar, baking powder and flour in a large bowl.
2. In a separate bowl, blend egg, oil, and milk all together until they mix completely.
3. Now, add the liquid mixture in step (ii) to the flour mixture. Stir until all the flour is dampened.
4. Add the blueberries and whisk gently
5. Cover the grill with cooking spray and heat to moderate heat
6. Pour 1/4 cup of batter on the hot grill and cook until it acquires a golden-brown color

7. Turn and cook the other side until it turns the same color.

8. It is prudent to serve while hot.

Nutritional Information per Serving

Serving Amount: 2 pancakes

Calories	158	Cholesterol	35mg
Total fat	4g	Sodium	240mg
Saturated fat	1g	Dietary fiber	4g
Total carbohydrate	28g	Added sugars	7g
Monounsaturated fat	2g	Trans fat	0g
Protein	6g		

Veggie egg bake

Number of Servings:6

Ingredients

- 1 cup frozen chopped spinach
- 4large eggs
- 4large egg whites
- 1cup skim milk
- 1 ½ teaspoons dry mustard
- 1 teaspoon dried rosemary or 1 tablespoon minced fresh rosemary
- 1/2 teaspoon salt-free herb-and-spice blend
- 1/4teaspoon ground black pepper
- 6slices whole-grain bread, crusts removed and cut into 1-inch cubes
- 1/4cup chopped onion
- 1/2 cup diced red pepper
- 4 ounces thinly sliced reduced-fat Swiss cheese

Instructions

1. Pre-heat the oven to about 190 C.
2. Sprinkle a 7 x11-inch glass baking dish with some cooking spray.
3. Put the spinach in a strainer and press it with the back of a spatula. This aims at removing excess liquid. After this, set it aside.

4. In a bowl, mix and stir milk, eggs, and egg whites. Also add dry mustard, spice blend, rosemary, and pepper (in small quantities) while still stirring.
5. Put the spinach, onion, bread, and red pepper in a separate large bowl.
6. Now, add the egg mixture and fling to coat.
7. Move the ingredients to a prepared baking dish and push down to compress. Cover the bowl with foil.
8. Put the bowl in the oven and bake until the eggs have set.
9. Uncover the ingredients and coat with a bit of cheese.
10. Resume baking for around 15 more minutes.
11. Transfer to a wire rack or tray and cool before serving.

Nutritional Information per Serving

Serving Amount: One piece

Calories	258	Sodium	465mg
Cholesterol	137mg	Dietary fiber	3g
Saturated fat	4g	Total carbohydrate	25g
Monounsaturated fat	2g	Added sugars	0g
Total fat	10g	Protein	17g

Overnight refrigerator oatmeal

Number of Servings: 1

Ingredients

- 1/3 cup skim milk or soy milk
- 1/4cup unsweetened applesauce
- 1/4cup old-fashioned rolled oats
- 1/4cup Greek low-fat plain yogurt
- 1/4cup diced apples
- 1 ½ teaspoons dried chia seeds
- 1/4teaspoon cinnamon

Instructions

1. Put all the ingredients in a mason jar.
2. Tighten the lid and shake to combine the contents.
3. Refrigerate overnight and eat the following morning whilst still cold.

Nutritional Information per Serving

Serving Amount: 1 cup

Calories 193 Sodium 89mg

Cholesterol	4mg	Dietary fiber	6g
Saturated fat	0g	Total carbohydrate	30g
Monounsaturated fat	1g	Added sugars	17g
Total fat	4g	Protein	11g
Trans fat	0g		

Spinach and mushroom frittata

Number of Servings:6

Ingredients

- 3cloves of garlic, minced
- 1 cup chopped onion
- 1 teaspoon olive oil
- 1/2-pound fresh mushrooms, sliced
- 1/2 teaspoon dried thyme
- 3-5 leaves of Fresh spinach
- 1tablespoon water
- Egg substitute equivalent to 10 eggs
- 1 tsp dried or fresh dill
- 1/4teaspoon black pepper
- 1/4 cup feta cheese

Instructions

1. Start by pre-heating the oven to around 175C.
2. Fry garlic and onion in olive oil in an ovenproof skillet for 5 minutes.
3. Then, add mushrooms and thyme and cook further for 5 minutes. Then remove the skillet from stove.
4. Chop the spinach leaves and squeeze out any liquid.
5. Put the spinach in another saucepan and add 1 tablespoon water. Cover and continue to cook until the spinach is wilted.

6.

7.   Beat the dill, pepper, and egg substitute in a large bowl

8.   Mix in the spinach-mushroom mixture and add some cheese.

9.   Abundantly spray a nonstick skillet with cooking spray and place it over moderate heat. After the skillet gets hot, pour in the egg mixture.

10. Place the mixture in the oven while uncovered and check every 5 minutes until the center of the frittata is slightly rigid.

11. After the frittata is done, place a large serving platter on the skillet and flip it over so that the frittata falls onto the plate.

12. Cut it into six to eight pieces and serve.

Nutritional Information per Serving

Serving Amount: 1 slice

Calories	106	Protein	4g
Cholesterol	6mg	Sodium	290mg
Saturated fat	1g	Dietary fiber	2g
Total fat	2g	Total sugar	3g
Monounsaturated fat	1g	Added sugars	0g
Trans fat	0g	Total carbohydrate	8g

Sweet potato soufflé

Number of Servings:6

Ingredients

- 1/2 cup panko breadcrumbs
- 4 cups mashed sweet potatoes
- 1/2 teaspoon unsalted butter
- 1 teaspoon chopped fresh thyme
- 1/4teaspoon salt and ground black pepper, mixed
- Pinch of ground nutmeg
- 1 ¾ cup skim milk
- 1 ½ tablespoons cornstarch
- 1/2 cup grated Gruyere cheese
- 3 egg whites

Instructions

1. Heat the oven to 190 C.
2. Sparingly cover 6 ramekins with cooking spray. In addition, sprinkle each with panko breadcrumbs.
3. Put the ramekins on a baking sheet.
4. Heat a medium-sized frying pan over moderate heat and add the butter, thyme, sweet potatoes, salt, pepper, and nutmeg.
5. In a relatively small bowl, mix milk and cornstarch to make a slurry and add it to the pan while whisking frequently until it comes to a light boil.

6. Decrease heat and stir in the cheese. After the cheese has melted, remove the mixture from heat and let it cool.

7. Beat the egg whites with an electric mixer until hard peaks form in a medium bowl.

8. Cautiously fold the sweet potato mixture into the egg whites.

9. Put equal amounts of the mixture into the ramekins and bake for about 20 minutes.

10. Remove from oven and serve while still hot.

Nutritional Information per Serving

Serving Amount: 1 slice

Calories	171	Protein	8g
Cholesterol	14mg	Dietary fiber	3g
Monounsaturated fat	1g	Total carbohydrate	26g
Total fat	4g	Sodium	273mg
Saturated fat	2g	Trans fat	0g
Total sugars	7g		

15 Lunch Recipes

Rice noodles with spring vegetables

Number of servings: 6

Ingredients

- 1package rice noodles
- 1tablespoon peanut oil
- 1tablespoon sesame oil
- 1tablespoon grated fresh ginger
- 2garlic cloves, finely chopped
- 2tablespoons low-sodium soy sauce
- 1cup small broccoli florets
- 1cup fresh bean sprouts
- 8cherry tomatoes, halved
- 1cup chopped fresh spinach
- 1 scallion, chopped
- Crushed red chili flakes (optional)

Instructions

1. Fill a relatively large pot three-fourths full with water and boil it.
2. Add the noodles and cook for around 5-6 minutes or according to the package instructions.
3. Remove and rinse the noodles with cold water and set aside.
4. In another frying pan, heat oils over moderate heat and add ginger and garlic. Stir while frying continues.

5. Add and stir the soy sauce and broccoli and carry on cooking for about 4 minutes. Add the remaining veggies and cooked noodles and toss until warmed.

6. Share the noodles among the warmed plates and cover each with crushed red chili flakes (optional).

7. Serve while hot.

Nutritional Information per Serving

Serving Amount: 1 ½ cups

Calories	205	Sodium	215mg
Cholesterol	0mg	Dietary fiber	1g
Total carbohydrate	37g	Total fat	5g
Saturated fat	1g	Added sugars	0g
Monounsaturated fat	2g	Protein	3g

Veggie pizza

Number of servings: 6

Ingredients

- One 12- to 15-inch refrigerated whole-wheat pizza crust
- 3/4cup spaghetti or pizza sauce
- 1 teaspoon salt-free Italian herb seasoning, divided
- 3/4 cup grated low-sodium, low-fat mozzarella

Pick three or more toppings from the list below:
- 1small onion, chopped
- 1large bell pepper, chopped
- 1/4 cup green or black olives, sliced
- 1 ½ cups sliced fresh mushrooms
- 1 cup broccoli florets
- 1 medium sliced zucchini
- 1sliced tomato

Instructions

1. Preheat the oven.
2. Place the outer layer of whole-wheat pizza crust on a baking stone.
3. Check the outer layer wrapper for baking temperature.

4. Use a cooking stick to evenly spread the sauce the outer layer.
5. Sprinkle the top with a 1/2teaspoonItalian herb seasoning. You can spread the cheese too.
6. Add the vegetables and sprinkle the remaining herb mixture.
7. Bake the pizza in line with the wrapper instructions.
8. Remove from the oven and cut into 6 wedges and serve.

Nutritional Information per Serving

Serving Amount: 1 slice (1/6th of pizza)

Calories	201	Total carbohydrate	28g
Cholesterol	8mg	Dietary fiber	5g
Total fat	5g	Sodium	405mg
Trans fat	0g	Saturated fat	3g
Protein	11g	Monounsaturated fat	2g

Smoky bean and mushroom cornucopias

Number of servings: 6

Ingredients

- 1tablespoon canola oil
- 2 cloves fresh garlic, minced
- 1/2 cup diced yellow onion
- 1/2 cup chopped Cremini mushrooms
- 1/4 cup diced bell pepper
- 1cup spinach, chopped
- 8ounces black beans, rinsed and drained
- 2 teaspoons chili powder
- 4 ounces fat-free sour cream
- 4 teaspoons liquid smoke
- 1/4 cup hot water
- Six 6 inch-diameter whole-wheat tortillas, cut in half
- 2teaspoons lime zest (optional garnish)

Instructions

1. Preheat the oven to 190 C.
2. Place some canola oil in fry pan and cook the garlic for about 1 minute.

3. Add onion and cook until it starts to turn golden brown. Add in mushrooms and cook further for about 2 minutes.
4. To these ingredients, add peppers and cook for 1 more minute then add in spinach, beans, and chili powder and remove from heat.
5. Allow the food to cool for 5 minutes and then fold in sour cream and liquid smoke.
6. To bring together all the ingredients, put the tortillas out on the counter and lightly brush the edges using some hot water.
7. Pinch the two edges together to form a seal using your finger. This will create the cornucopia shell.
8. Position the rolled tortilla shell on a baking sheet lined by a parchment paper.
9. After filling tortillas with stuffing, bake for around 20-25 minutes
10. Immediately serve with a favorite salsa.

Nutritional Information per Serving

Serving Amount: 2 pieces

Calories	206	Total carbohydrate	30g
Saturated fat	2g	Total f	7g
Monounsaturated fat	3g	Sodium	343g
Cholesterol	0mg	Dietary fiber	7g
Protein	8g	Added sugars	4g
Trans fat	0g		

Vegetarian kebabs

Number of servings: 2

Ingredients

- 8 cherry tomatoes
- 8 button mushrooms
- 1 small zucchini, sliced into 8 pieces
- 1 red onion, cut into 4 wedges
- 1 green bell pepper, seeded and cut into 4pieces
- 1 red bell pepper, seeded and cut into 4pieces
- 1/2 cup fat-free Italian dressing
- 1/2 cup brown rice
- 1 cup water
- 4 wooden skewers, soaked in water for 30 minutes, or metal skewers

Instructions

1. Put the zucchini, onion, tomatoes, mushrooms, and peppers in a sealed plastic bag. Add the Italian dressing and gently shake to cover the vegetables evenly.
2. Put aside the vegetables for not less than 10 minutes.
3. Combine the rice and water in a saucepan over extreme heat to boil. Slowly decrease heat, cover but simmer until the water is absorbed and the rice is

tender. Transfer the cooked rice into a small bowl and cover to keep warm.

4. Set up a hot fire in a charcoal grill or heat a gas grill. Away from the heat source, sparingly cover the grill rack with cooking spray and position the cooking rack about 4 to 6 inches from the heat source.

5. Thread 2 mushrooms, 2 zucchini slices, 2 tomatoes, 1 onion wedge, and 1 green and red pepper slice onto each skewer.

6. Put the kebabs on the grill rack and baste with leftover marinade.

7. Cook for about 5 to 8 minutes until the vegetables are tender.

8. Share the rice onto 2 plates.

9. Cover the rice with 2-3 kebabs and serve while still hot.

Nutritional Information per Serving

Serving Amount: 2 kebabs and about ¾ cup of rice

Calories	335	Protein	10g
Cholesterol	1mg	Dietary fiber	8g
Total fat	3g	Total carbohydrate	67g
Monounsaturated fat	0.5g	Sodium	335mg
Trans fat	0g	Added sugars	0g
Saturated fat	0.5g		

Turkey bean soup

Number of servings: 4

Ingredients

- 1-pound ground turkey breast
- 2medium onions, chopped
- 2stalks celery, chopped
- 1clove garlic, minced
- 1/4 cup ketchup
- 1can unsalted diced tomatoes
- 3 cubes low-sodium chicken bouillon
- 7 cups water
- 1 ½ teaspoons dried basil
- 1/4 teaspoon ground black pepper
- 2cups shredded cabbage
- 1 can of unsalted cannellini beans, rinsed and drained

Instructions

1. Cook the ground turkey, onion, celery, and garlic in a large saucepan until the vegetables are softened and the whole turkey is properly cooked.
2. Add the bouillon, water, basil, pepper, ketchup, tomatoes, beans, and cabbage.
3. Ensure you boil and afterward reduce the heat.
4. Cover for 30 minutes.
5. Serve while hot.

Nutritional Information per Serving

Serving Amount: 3 ½ cups

Calories	242	Sodium	204mg
Total fat	2g	Total carbohydrate	30g
Saturated fat	Less than 1g	Dietary fiber	10g
Trans fat	0g	Added sugars	0g
Cholesterol	37mg	Protein	26g

Turkey and broccoli crepes

Number of servings: Four

Ingredients

- 2cups chopped broccoli
- 4pre-packaged crepes, 8 inches each
- 4ounces reduced-sodium turkey breast, sliced
- 1/2cup finely shredded reduced-fat Colby jack cheese

Instructions

1. Pre-heat the oven to 175 C.
2. Evenly coat a baking dish using some cooking spray.
3. Boil 1 inch of water in a pot fitted with a steamer basket.
4. After the water has boiled, add the broccoli and cover to steam 5 to 7 minutes until tender.
5. Heat the crepes in the microwave for about 1 minute or in line with package instructions.
6. Place 1/4 turkey, 1/4 cup steamed broccoli, and 2 tablespoons cheese on each crepe.
7. Place seam-side down and turn up in the prepared baking dish.
8. Continue to bake for about 5 minutes until all the cheese melts.
9. Serve while hot.

Nutritional Information per Serving

Serving Amount: 1 crepe

Calories	223	Sodium	200mg
Saturated fat	4g	Total carbohydrate	23g
Monounsaturated fat	1g	Dietary fiber	3g
Total fat	7g	Total sugars	14g
Cholesterol	47mg	Added sugars	0g
Protein	17g		

Tomato basil pesto sauce

Number of servings: 10 - 15

Ingredients

- 1/4 cup olive oil
- 4 garlic cloves, minced
- 1/4 cup red wine vinegar
- 8 cups diced Roma tomatoes
- 1/2 cup tomato paste
- 12 fresh basil leaves, chopped
- 1 tablespoon sugar
- 1/2 teaspoon salt
- 1/4 teaspoon ground pepper
- 1/2 cup grated Parmesan cheese

Instructions

1. Heat a relatively large saucepan with medium-low heat and add the oil.
2. When the oil is heated, add the garlic and sauté until it appears golden brown in color and add the vinegar and fry for 2 more minutes.
3. Stir in the tomato paste, basil, sugar, tomatoes, pepper, and salt.
4. Simmer the mixture while stirring until the tomatoes break down.

5. Withdraw the frying pan from the heat and let it cool. Blend the sauce and cheese in a food processor until it becomes completely smooth.

6. Add seasoning and taste the sauce to acquire the desired flavor.

Nutritional Information per Serving

Serving Amount: ½ cup

Calories	85	Sodium	344mg
Total fat	4g	Total carbohydrate	8g
Saturated fat	1g	Dietary fiber	1g
Monounsaturated fat	3g	Total sugars	2g
Cholesterol	2mg	Protein	2g
Trans fat	0g		

Vegetable lasagna roll-ups

Number of servings: 6

Ingredients

Lasagna roll-ups:

- 6 whole-wheat lasagna noodles
- 1 teaspoon olive oil
- 3/4 cup chopped mushrooms
- 3/4 cup chopped onions
- 1 tablespoon chopped fresh garlic
- 1/4 cup Burgundy wine
- 1 cup chopped zucchini
- 3/4 cup chopped beefsteak tomatoes
- 1/2 cup part-skim ricotta cheese
- 3/4 cup shredded part-skim mozzarella cheese
- 1/4 cup basil pesto mayo
- 1/4 cup chopped red bell pepper

Pesto mayonnaise:

- 1 cup fresh basil leaves
- 1/4 cup pumpkin seeds
- 1/4 cup fresh Parmesan cheese
- 3 cloves garlic, minced
- 1/2 teaspoon kosher salt
- 1 cup reduced-fat mayonnaise

Instructions

1. Place basil leaves, Parmesan, garlic, salt and pumpkin seeds in a food processor in order to make the pesto spread.
2. Process ingredients while adding mayonnaise and pulse until they are well-blended and fairly smooth and set aside.
3. At this juncture, heat oven to 175 C.
4. Lightly smear a baking dish with cooking spray.
5. Boil some water in a large pot and add lasagna noodles and cook until they are done. Drain the water and set aside the noodles.
6. Heat the olive oil in a relatively large nonstick fry pan and add the onions, garlic, mushrooms, and fry for 3 minutes.
7. Add some wine and cook until all of the wine has been reduced down. Moreover, add the zucchini and tomatoes, continue frying further for 3 to 5 minutes.
8. When tender, remove the frying pan from heat and set aside.
9. Now, add ricotta and 1/4 cup of the mozzarella.
10. Set the cooked lasagna noodles in the baking dish and lightly cover them with cooking spray.
11. Place 1/2cup of the vegetable mixture at the end of each noodle and roll up.
12. Sprinkle the pesto mayonnaise over the noodles and cover with kitchen foil to bake for about 25 minutes more.
13. Remove the foil and sprinkle with remaining mozzarella and chopped peppers.

14. Bake until all the cheese is melted. This will around 3 minutes.
15. Serve immediately

Nutritional Information per Serving

Serving Amount: 1 roll-up

Calories	227	Sodium	291mg
Saturated fat	3g	Total fat	9g
Cholesterol	19mg	Trans fat	0g
Total carbohydrate	24g	Dietary fiber	5g
Monounsaturated fat	3g	Total sugars	4g
Protein	12g		

Pita pizza

Number of servings: 2

Ingredients

- 2whole-wheat pita loaves
- 1/2cup marinara
- 1/2 cup diced red onion
- 1/4 cup sliced button mushrooms
- 1/4 cup diced pineapple
- 1/4 cup diced bell pepper
- 6tablespoons part-skim mozzarella cheese
- 1/4cup reduced-fat feta cheese
- 2teaspoons turkey bacon bits

Instructions

1. Heat the oven to 190 C.
2. Lightly coat a baking sheet using some cooking spray.
3. Put the pitas on the baking sheet and spread the marinara over them.
4. Cover the pizzas with equal amounts of onion, pineapple, peppers and mushrooms and sprinkle with cheeses and bacon bits.
5. Bake until all the cheese is golden brown in color.
6. Withdraw from the heat and serve.

Nutritional Information per Serving

Serving Amount: 1 pizza

Calories	324	Sodium	820mg
Total fat	17g	Protein	17g
Monounsaturated fat	1g	Total carbohydrate	48g
Cholesterol	21mg	Total sugars	9g
Saturated fat	3g	Dietary fiber	4g
Trans fat	0g		

Marinated Portobello mushrooms with provolone

Number of servings: 2

Ingredients

- 2 Portobello mushrooms, stemmed and wiped clean
- 1/2cup balsamic vinegar
- 1 tablespoon brown sugar
- 1/4 teaspoon dried rosemary
- One teaspoon minced garlic
- 1/4 cup grated provolone cheese

Instructions

1. Set up and heat a grill.
2. Position the rack 4 inches from the heat source and lightly cover a glass baking dish with cooking spray.
3. Place the mushrooms in the dish
4. In a medium-sized bowl whisk together the rosemary, vinegar, brown sugar, and garlic.
5. Pour the mixture over the mushrooms and set aside for 5 to 10 minutes to marinate.
6. Broil the mushrooms while still turning until they are tender on each side.
7. Sprinkle grated cheese over each mushroom and continue to grill until all the cheese melts.
8. Transfer to individual plates and serve immediately.

Nutritional Information per Serving

Serving Amount: 1 mushroom

Calories	112	Sodium	140mg
Cholesterol	10mg	Dietary fiber	1g
Total fat	4g	Added sugars	4g
Saturated fat	2g	Total sugars	11g
Monounsaturated fat	1g	Total carbohydrate	13g
Protein	6g		

Hot ham and cheese sandwiches with mushrooms

Number of servings: 2

Ingredients

- 2tablespoons fat-free mayonnaise
- 2teaspoons Dijon mustard
- 2slices rye bread
- 4ounces thinly sliced ham
- 2slices red onion
- 1can sliced mushrooms, drained and patted dry
- 2ounces low-fat Swiss cheese, thinly sliced

Instructions

1. Heat the grill to a high temperature and position the rack about 4 inches from the heat source.
2. Sparingly smear a baking sheet using cooking spray.
3. Mix the mayonnaise and mustard in a small bowl.
4. Put the slices of bread on the prepared baking sheet.
5. Spread half of the mayonnaise mixture on each slice and cover each with halfof the mushrooms, 1-ounce cheese, 2 ounces ham, and 1 slice onions.
6. For about 3 minutes, broil the open-faced sandwiches until the cheese is fully melted and slightly browned.
7. Serve while hot.

Nutritional Information per Serving

Serving Amount: 1 open-faced sandwich

Calories	229	Total carbohydrate	25g
Saturated fat	2g	Sodium	1195mg
Total fat	5g	Dietary fiber	4g
Monounsaturated fat	2g	Protein	21g
Cholesterol	36mg	Added sugars	0g
Trans fat	0g	Total sugars	7g

Hearty turkey chili

Number of servings:8

Ingredients

- 2cups chopped zucchini
- 1teaspoon olive oil
- 1cup chopped onion
- 2cups chopped celery
- 1cup chopped bell peppers
- 2teaspoons chopped fresh garlic
- 1pound chopped cooked turkey
- 1 ½ tablespoons chili powder
- 1teaspoon cumin seed
- 2cups diced canned tomatoes, no-salt-added variety
- 4 cups canned kidney beans, rinsed and drained
- 2cups low-sodium vegetable broth
- 1teaspoon brown sugar

Instructions

1. Preheat the oven to 245 C.
2. Spray a glass baking dish with cooking spray and arrange the zucchini in a single layer.
3. Bake for 8 to 10 minutes.
4. While the zucchini is roasting, add the oil and chopped onions into a Dutch oven or soup pot.

5. Fry the mixture over low heat until the onions are browned.
6. Add the celery and peppers and continue to fry.
7. Add garlic, chili, powder, cumin seed, and turkey
8. Wrap the baking dish and simmer for about 5 minutes.
9. Stir in the tomatoes, vegetable broth, brown sugar, zucchini, and the roasted kidney beans.
10. Wrap the baking dish and simmer for 15 minutes and scoop into warmed individual bowls.
11. Serve immediately.

Nutritional Information per Serving

Serving Amount: 1 ½ cups

Calories	252	Sodium	178mg
Total fat	4g	Total carbohydrate	28g
Cholesterol	57mg	Dietary fiber	8g
Saturated fat	1g	Added sugars	0.5g
Protein	26g	Monounsaturated fat	2g

Rice and beans salad

Number of servings: 5 - 10

Ingredients

- 1 ½ cups uncooked brown rice
- 3cups water
- 1/2 cup chopped fresh parsley
- 1/2 cup chopped shallots or spring onions
- 15-ounce can unsalted garbanzo beans, rinsed and drained
- 15-ounce can unsalted dark kidney beans, rinsed and drained
- 1/4 cup olive oil
- 1/2 cup rice vinegar, according to your taste

Instructions

1. Put rice and water into pot.
2. Cover and cook for about 45 to 50 minutes over medium heat until rice is tender.
3. Allow the rice to cool to room temperature.
4. Stir in the remaining ingredients.
5. Serve with beans.

Nutritional Information per Serving

Serving Amount: 3/4cup

Calories	227	Total carbohydrate	34g
Saturated fat	1g	Dietary fiber	5g
Cholesterol	0mg	Sodium	110mg
Total fat	7g	Protein	7g
Monounsaturated fat	4g	Total sugars	3g
Trans fat	0g	Added sugars	0g

Steak with Chimichurri Sauce

Number of servings: 4

Ingredients

- 1-pound skirt steak
- 1/2cup red wine vinegar
- 1/2 cup olive oil
- 2 shallots
- 4 garlic cloves
- 1/2 bunch cilantro leaves
- 2 tablespoons parsley
- 1 tablespoon fresh oregano
- 1 teaspoon crushed red pepper flakes
- 1/2 teaspoon sugar
- 1/4 teaspoon kosher salt

Instructions

1. Trim off the excess fat and tissue from skirt steak meat.
2. Combine oil, shallots, parsley, vinegar, oregano, crushed pepper flakes, garlic, cilantro, and sugar in a food processor.
3. The marinade should be a little thick and very green once it is fully blended.
4. Put the marinade in a bowl together with the steak and let marinate for the night in the refrigerator.

5. Heat the grill high and remove the meat from the refrigerator to let it come to room temperature for about 20 minutes.
6. Place the meat on a hot grill for about 2-4 minutes to let grill marks to be made before flipping.
7. After both sides are fully cooked, remove the meat from heat and put it on a cutting board.
8. Cut the steak into 2-inch thick pieces and then turn and cut against the grain.
9. Shake over with a bit of salt and serve while hot.

Nutritional Information per Serving

Serving Amount: 4 ounces

Calories	333	Total carbohydrate	4g
Cholesterol1	104mg	Sodium	209mg
Saturated fat	6g	Dietary fiber	1g
Total fat	20g	Added sugars	1g
Monounsaturated fat	10g	Protein	34g
Trans fat	1g		

Grilled turkey burger

Number of servings: 4

Ingredients

- 1-pound ground turkey breast
- 1/4cup dried bread crumbs
- 1/4 cup chopped onion
- 2 tablespoons fresh parsley, chopped
- 1 ½ tablespoons Worcestershire sauce
- 1teaspoon Tabasco (hot) sauce
- 4whole-grain buns
- 4slices tomato
- 4slices red onion
- 2Bibb lettuce leaves, halved
- 4tablespoons ketchup

Instructions

1. Mix the dried bread crumbs, turkey breast, parsley, chopped onion, and hot sauce and Worcestershire sauce in a large bowl.
2. Divide turkey mixture into 4 equal portions and make them into pies.
3. Prepare a hot fire in a charcoal grill and put a pan sprinkled with cooking spray a bit away from the heat source. By doing so the cooking rack will be 4 to 6 inches from the heat source.

4. Grill burgers until they are browned on both sides and heated through for about 7 minutes a side.

5. Serve each burger on a bun topped with 1 tomato, 1/2 sliced lettuce leave, a dollop of ketchup, and 1 onion slice.

Nutritional Information per Serving

Serving Amount: 1 burger

Calories	292	Sodium	484mg
Cholesterol	45mg	Dietary fiber	3g
Monounsaturated fat	1g	Total carbohydrate	28g
Saturated fat	1g	Protein	36g
Trans fat	0g	Added sugars	0g
Total fat	4g		

15 Dinner Recipes

Fried rice

Number of servings: 4

Ingredients

- 2cups cooked brown rice
- 3tablespoons peanut oil
- 4green onions with tops
- 2carrots, finely chopped
- 1/2 finely chopped green bell pepper
- 1/2 frozen peas
- 1egg
- 2tablespoons low-sodium soy sauce
- 1tablespoon sesame oil
- 1/4cup chopped parsley

Instructions

1. Put some peanut oil in a large, heavy skillet.
2. Heat the peanut oil over medium-high heat.
3. Add cooked rice and fry until it turns golden brown. On top of these ingredients, add carrots, green pepper, green onions, and peas.
4. For about 5 minutes, continue frying while stirring until vegetables turn tender.
5. Scoop out a circle at the center of the skillet by shoving the vegetables and rice to the sides.

6. Smash the egg into the hollow space and cook while stirring to mix up the eggs as they cook.
7. After the eggs completely cook, stir them into the rice mixture.
8. Sparingly sprinkle the ingredients with soy sauce, sesame oil, and chopped parsley.
9. Serve immediately.

Nutritional Information per Serving

Serving Amount: 1.5 cups

Calories	279	Total carbohydrate	31g
Saturated fat	3g	Sodium	116mg
Monounsaturated fat	7g	Dietary fiber	4mg
Cholesterol	47g	Protein	6g
Total fat	16g	Added sugars	0g

Curried carrot soup

Number of servings: 6

Ingredients

- 1tablespoon olive oil
- 1 teaspoon mustard seed
- 1/2 cup yellow onion, chopped
- 1 pound carrots, peeled and cut into 1/2-inch pieces
- 1 tablespoon plus 1teaspoon peeled and chopped fresh ginger
- 1/2 jalapeño, seeded
- 2teaspoons curry powder
- 2cups low-sodium chicken stock, vegetable stock or broth
- 1/4 cup chopped fresh cilantro, plus leaves for garnish
- 2tablespoons fresh lime juice
- 1/2teaspoon salt
- 3tablespoons low-fat sour cream or fat-free plain yogurt
- Grated zest of 1lime

Instructions

1. Heat the olive oil over medium heat in a large saucepan and add the mustard seed.

2. When the seeds start to crack, add the onion and fry for about 4 minutes until it becomes soft and translucent.
3. Now, add the carrots, jalapeño, curry powder, and ginger and continue frying for about 3 minutes or until the seasonings become aromatic.
4. Add 3 cups of the stock and increase the heat to boil.
5. Decrease the heat to medium-low and simmer the carrots for about 6 minutes until they appear tender.
6. In a blender, process the soups in small batches until smooth and return to the saucepan. Note that the soup will become hot within 5 minutes.
7. Note that the blender should be filled no more than one-third full to evade burns.
8. Stir in the remaining 2 cups of stock and return the soup to medium heat and reheat gently.
9. Before serving, stir in the chopped cilantro and lime juice.
10. If desired, season the ingredients with the salt and scoop into warmed individual bowls.
11. Garnish with a sprinkle of warm yogurt, lime zest, and cilantro leaves and serve.

Nutritional Information per Serving

Serving Amount: 1.5 cups

Calories	104	Total carbohydrate	12g
Saturated fat	1g	Sodium	116mg

Monounsaturated fat	2g	Dietary fiber	2.5g
Protein	5g	Trans fat	0g
Total fat	4g	Added sugars	0g
Total sugar	4g	Cholesterol	1mg

Turkey breast burgers

Number of servings: 2

Ingredients

- 1/2-pound ground turkey breast
- 1/2cup chopped onion
- 1/2tablespoons chopped fresh cilantro
- 1/2teaspoon garlic powder
- 1/2teaspoon onion powder
- 1/2teaspoon cumin
- 1/2teaspoon salt
- 1/4teaspoon black pepper
- 1 egg
- 2 whole-grain buns

Instructions

1. Set up the grill and heat a skillet to medium heat.
2. Mix the turkey breast, cilantro, garlic powder, onion, onion powder, cumin, eggs, and pepper in a medium-sized bowl.
3. Divide the mixture into two 4-ounce patties
4. Smear the cooking surface with cooking spray and place the patties on top.
5. Cook for about 5 minutes while turning each side to ensure that each side gets a golden-brown color.

6. Withdraw the patties from heat and let them rest until about 75 C.

7. Serve on whole-grain buns.

Nutritional Information per Serving

Serving Amount: 1 patty and 1 whole-grain bun

Calories	289	Sodium	640mg
Cholesterol	148mg	Total carbohydrate	28g
Saturated fat	2g	Dietary fiber	5g
Total fat	6g	Trans fat	0g
Monounsaturated fat	1g	Total sugars	2g
Protein	36g		

Paella with chicken, leeks, and tarragon

Number of servings: 4

Ingredients

- 1teaspoon extra-virgin olive oil
- 1small onion, sliced
- 2leeks (whites only), thinly sliced
- 3garlic cloves, minced
- 1-pound boneless, skinless chicken breast, (Cut into strips 1/2-inch wide and 10 cm long)
- 2large tomatoes, chopped
- 1red pepper, sliced
- 2/3 cup long-grain brown rice
- 1teaspoon tarragon, or to taste
- 2cups fat-free, unsalted chicken broth
- 1cup frozen peas
- 1/4cup chopped fresh parsley (optional)
- 1lemon, cut into 4 wedges(optional)

Instructions

1. Heat olive oil under medium heat in a large and nonstick frying pan.
2. When the oil gets hot, add the leeks, garlic, onions, and chicken strips.

3. Sauté for about 5 minutes until the vegetables are translucent and chicken gets slightly browned.
4. Now, add the red pepper slices and tomatoes and continue to fry for another 5 minutes.
5. Add rice, tarragon, and broth and mix thoroughly and continue to cook until it boils.
6. Decrease the heat and simmer about 10 minutes whilst the ingredients are uncovered.
7. Add the peas and stir together with other ingredients and continue to simmer uncovered for around 45 to 60 minutes or until broth is absorbed and the rice is tender.
8. Divide in individual plates to serve.
9. You can decorate each plate with 1 tablespoon parsley and 1 lemon wedge.

Nutritional Information per Serving

Serving Amount: 2 cups rice and vegetables and 4 ounces chicken

Calories	378	Sodium	182mg
Cholesterol	82mg	Total carbohydrate	46g
Saturated fat	1g	Dietary fiber	7g
Total fat	6g	Added sugars	0g
Monounsaturated fat	2g	Protein	35g

Braised celery root

Number of servings: 6

Ingredients

- 1cup vegetable stock or broth
- 1celery root (celeriac), about 3 cups, peeled and diced
- 1/4cup sour cream
- 1teaspoon Dijon mustard
- 1/4teaspoon salt
- 1/4teaspoon freshly ground black pepper
- 2teaspoons fresh thyme leaves

Instructions

1. Bring the stock to a boil over high heat in a relatively large saucepan and add the celery root while stirring.
2. Reduce the heat to low when the stock returns to a boil.
3. Cover and simmer until the celery root is tender. Ensure you stir occasionally.
4. Using a slotted spoon, move the celery root to a bowl and cover to keep warm.
5. Increase the heat under the saucepan and make the cooking liquid to boil.
6. Cook uncovered for about 5 minutes until reduced to 1 tablespoon

7. Withdraw from the heat and beat in the sour cream, mustard, salt and pepper mixture.
8. Now, add the celery root and thyme to the sauce and stir over medium heat.
9. Transfer everything to a warmed serving dish.
10. Serve immediately.

Nutritional Information per Serving

Serving Amount: 1/2 cup

Calories	54	Protein	2g
Cholesterol	4mg	Dietary fiber	1g
Monounsaturated fat	0g	Sodium	206mg
Trans fat	0g	Total carbohydrate	7g
Saturated fat	1g	Total sugars	1.5g
Total fat	2g	Added sugars	0g

Broccoli with garlic and lemon

Number of servings: 2

Ingredients

- 4cups broccoli florets
- 1teaspoon olive oil
- 1tablespoon minced garlic
- 1teaspoon lemon zest
- 1/4teaspoon kosher salt
- 1/4 teaspoon ground black pepper

Instructions

1. Boil1 cup of water in a small saucepan.
2. Add the broccoli to the boiling water and cook until tender.
3. Drain broccoli.
4. Heat the oil in a small sauté pan over a medium-high flame.
5. Add the garlic and fry for just 30 seconds and add lemon zest, broccoli, salt and pepper.
6. Mix thoroughly and serve.

Nutritional Information per Serving

Serving Amount: 1 cup

Calories	45	Protein	3g
Cholesterol	0mg	Dietary fiber	3g
Monounsaturated fat	1g	Sodium	153mg
Trans fat	0g	Total sugars	2g
Total fat	1g	Total carbohydrate	7g
Saturated fat	0g		

Brussels sprouts with shallots and lemon

Number of servings: 4

Ingredients

- 3 teaspoons extra-virgin olive oil, divided
- 3shallots, thinly sliced (about 3 tablespoons)
- 1/4teaspoon salt, divided
- 1-pound Brussels sprouts, trimmed and cut into quarters
- 1/2cup no-salt-added vegetable stock or broth
- 1/4 teaspoon finely grated lemon zest
- 1tablespoon fresh lemon juice
- 1/4teaspoon freshly ground black pepper

Instructions

1. In a large and nonstick sauté pan, heat 2 teaspoons of the olive oil under medium heat.
2. Add the shallots and fry for about 6 minutes until soft and lightly golden.
3. Add 1/8 teaspoon salt and stir.
4. Transfer these ingredients to a bowl and set aside.
5. Heat the remaining 1 teaspoon olive oil over medium heat in the same frying pan.
6. Add the Brussels sprouts and continue frying until they start to brown.

7. Add the vegetable stock and simmer uncovered until the Brussels sprouts are tender.
8. Put back the shallots into the pan and stir with the 1/8 teaspoon salt, the lemon zest and juice, and the pepper.
9. Serve immediately while hot.

Nutritional Information per Serving

Serving Amount: 1/4cup

Calories	104	Protein	5g
Cholesterol	0mg	Total sugar	3g
Monounsaturated fat	2g	Total carbohydrate	12g
Saturated fat	1g	Dietary fiber	5g
Total fat	4g	Sodium	191mg
Trans fat	0g	Added sugars	0g

Green beans with red pepper and garlic

Number of servings: 6

Ingredients

- 1-pound green beans, stems trimmed
- 2teaspoons olive oil
- 1red bell pepper, seeded and cut into thin slices
- 1/2teaspoon chili paste or red pepper flakes
- 1clove garlic, finely chopped
- 1teaspoon sesame oil
- 1/2 teaspoon salt
- 1/4 teaspoon freshly ground black pepper

Instructions

1. Cut the beans into 2-inch slices.
2. Add water to a large sauce pan until three-fourths full and boil.
3. Now, add the beans and cook until they turn bright green and are tender-crunchy.
4. Drain the beans and immerse them into a bowl of ice water. Drain again and put aside.
5. Heat the olive oil over medium heat in a large frying pan and add the bell pepper. Toss and stir for about 1 minute.
6. Add beans and fry for 1 more minute.

7. Add chili paste and garlic and stir for 1 minute.
8. Sprinkle with the sesame oil and season with the salt and pepper.
9. Serve while hot.

Nutritional Information per Serving

Serving Amount: 3/4cup

Calories54	54	Sodium	202mg
Cholesterol0 mg	0mg	Protein	2g
Dietary fiber2 g	2g	Monounsaturated fat	1g
Total fat2 g	2g	Added sugars	0g
Trans fat0 g	0g	Total carbohydrate	7g
Saturated fat<1 g	Less than 1g		

Grilled chicken salad with olives and oranges

Number of servings: 4

Ingredients

For the dressing:

- 1/2cup red wine vinegar
- 4 garlic cloves, minced
- 1tablespoon extra-virgin olive oil
- 1tablespoon finely chopped red onion
- 1tablespoon finely chopped celery
- Cracked black pepper, to taste

For the salad:

- 4boneless, skinless chicken breasts, each 4 ounces
- atleast 6garlic cloves
- 8cups leaf lettuce, washed and dried
- 16large ripe (black) olives
- 2navel oranges, peeled and sliced

Instructions

1. Combine 2 garlic, olive oil, the vinegar, onion, pepper and celery in a small bowl.
2. Stir to mix evenly to make the dressing and then cover and refrigerate until needed.
3. Set up a charcoal grill with a hot fire and place the grill smeared with cooking spray about 4-6 inches away from the sauce.
4. Sprinkle the chicken breasts using 2 or 3 garlic cloves.
5. Broil the chicken until browned for about 5 minutes on each side.
6. Move the chicken to a chopping board and let it to cool for 5 minutes before slicing into strips.
7. Set up four plates so that each has 2 cups lettuce, 4 olives, and 1/4 of the sliced oranges
8. Top each plate with 1 chicken breast cut into strips and sprinkle with the refrigerated dressing.
9. Serve immediately.

Nutritional Information per Serving

Serving Amount: 2 cups lettuce plus toppings

Calories	237	Dietary fiber	3g
Monounsaturated fat	5g	Total carbohydrate	12g
Cholesterol	83mg	Protein	27g
Saturated fat	1g	Added sugars	0g
Total fat	9g	Sodium	199mg

Chicken Caesar pitas

Number of servings: 2

Ingredients

- 1can (5 ounces) chunky white meat chicken packed in water, drained
- 3/4cup chopped romaine lettuce
- 1Roma tomato, chopped
- 1/4cup grated fresh Parmesan cheese
- 1/3 cup fat-free Caesar dressing
- 1whole-wheat pita bread, cut in half

Instructions

1. Mix the chicken, Parmesan cheese, tomato, lettuce, and Caesar dressing in a small bowl.
2. Ensure all ingredients are mixed evenly.
3. Cover and place in the fridge for about 10 – to 15 minutes.
4. Squeeze the chicken mixture into the pita bread halves and serve immediately

Nutritional Information per Serving

Serving Amount: 1 pita half

Calories	219	Sodium	1047mg
Cholesterol	33mg	Protein	18g
Total fat	5g	Total carbohydrate	24g
Monounsaturated fat	1g	Dietary fiber	4g
Saturated fat	3g		

Brown rice pilaf

Number of servings: 8

Ingredients

- 1 ¼ cups dark brown rice, rinsed and drained
- 2 cups water
- 3/4 teaspoon salt
- 1/4 teaspoon saffron threads or ground turmeric
- 1/2 teaspoon grated orange zest
- 3 tablespoons fresh orange juice
- 1 ½ tablespoons pistachio oil or canola oil
- 1/4 cup chopped pistachio nuts
- 1/4 cup dried apricots, chopped

Instructions

1. Combine 1/4 teaspoon of the salt, rice, saffron, and water in a saucepan placed over high heat.
2. Wait until it starts to boil and reduce the heat to low,
3. Cover and simmer until all the water is soaked up and the rice is tender.
4. Transfer the rice to a large bowl and cover with foil to keep warm.
5. In a relatively small bowl, combine the remaining 1/2 teaspoon salt, orange zest and juice, and oil.
6. Whisk and ensure that all ingredients are completely blended.

7. Now, gently pour the orange mixture over the warm rice and add the nuts and apricots.

8. Toss gently to mix. Coat and serve immediately.

Nutritional Information per Serving

Serving Amount: 1/2cup

Calories	153	Protein	3g
Cholesterol	0mg	Sodium	222mg
Saturated fat	1g	Dietary fiber	2g
Total fat	5g	Total carbohydrate	24g
Monounsaturated fat	3g		

Beef and vegetable kebabs

Number of servings: 2

Ingredients

- 1/2 cup brown rice
- 2 cups water
- 4 ounces top sirloin (choice)
- 4 tablespoons fat-free Italian dressing
- 1 green pepper, seeded and cut into 4 pieces
- 4 cherry tomatoes
- 1small onion, cut into 4 wedges
- 2wooden skewers, soaked in water for 30 minutes, or metal skewers

Instructions

1. In a relatively large pot, combine the rice and water and bring to a boil.
2. Reduce the heat to low and simmer while covered until all the water is absorbed and the rice is tender.
3. Transfer the rice to a small bowl and cover with foil to keep warm.
4. Cut the meat into 4 equal portions and place in a small bowl.
5. Sprinkle the Italian dressing over the top of the meat.
6. Put the meat in the freezer for at least 20 minutes to marinate.

7. Prepare a hot fire in a charcoal grill, smear the grill rack with cooking spray and place it away from the heat.
8. Thread 2 cubes of meat, 2 green pepper pieces, 2 cherry tomatoes, and 2 onion wedges onto each skewer and place the kebabs on the grill rack.
9. Grill the kebabs for about 5 to 10 minutes while turning to cook all sides
10. Divide the rice onto individual plates and top with 1 kebab.
11. Serve immediately.

Nutritional Information per Serving

Serving Amount: 1 kebab and 3/4cup rice

Calories	300	Total carbohydrate	49g
Saturated fat	1g	Dietary fiber	4g
Total fat	3g	Sodium	450 mg
Cholesterol	39 mg	Protein	18g
Monounsaturated fat	1g	Added sugars	0g

Roasted turkey with balsamic sauce

Number of servings: 7 - 10

Ingredients

For the turkey:

- 1 whole turkey
- 1 tablespoon olive oil
- 4 sprigs fresh rosemary
- 3-4 cloves garlic
- 1/2 cup water

For the sauce:

- 1 cup balsamic vinegar
- 1 cup defatted pan drippings
- 3 tablespoons brown sugar

Instructions

1. Pre-heat the oven to 165 C.
2. Clean the turkey inside and out with flowing water and then dry the outside by patting with paper towels.
3. Put the turkey breast-side up on a rack in a boiling pan

4. Smear the turkey with the oil and spray a bit on the rosemary and garlic cloves.

5. Place all the remaining rosemary and garlic inside the turkey carcass.

6. Tie the legs together with a loose knot and place into the middle of the oven.

7. Dry for about an hour until the skin is light brown.

8. Withdraw the turkey from the oven and cover it with foil to prevent overcooking and continue roasting for about 3 hours.

9. Turkey is okay if the thigh is pierced deeply with a toothpick and juices run clear

10. Remove the turkey from the oven set it up in a position that can allow juices to settle in the meat.

11. Add about half a cup of water and stir to scratch up browned bits. Pour the pan drippings into a gravy separator but reserve 1 cup of defatted pan drippings as sauce.

12. To make the sauce, put the vinegar, defatted pan drippings, and brown sugar in a pan and stir together.

13. Moderately heat the sauce until the aroma is released. Ensure that the sauce does not boil.

14. Slice the turkey and sprinkle with the warmed brown sugar sauce.

15. Serve immediately while still hot.

Nutritional Information per Serving

Serving Amount: 5 ounces light and dark meat

Calories	280	Sodium	154mg
Total fat	8g	Total carbohydrate	9g
Monounsaturated fat	3g	Added sugars	3g
Cholesterol	150mg	Protein	43g
Saturated fat	2g		

Chicken adobo soup with bok choy

Number of servings: 4

Ingredients

- 1/3 cup reduced-sodium soy sauce
- 1/3 cup rice vinegar
- 2 garlic cloves, sliced
- 1bay leaf
- 1teaspoon olive oil
- 1/2 yellow onion, chopped
- One and a Half cups skinned and shredded roasted or boiled chicken breast meat
- 1/2 cup uncooked whole-wheat couscous or 1 cup cooked brown rice
- 1/2 pound baby bok choy, halved lengthwise and sliced crosswise Half -inch wide
- 2 green onions, including tender green tops, thinly sliced

Instructions

1. In a small pan, mix the vinegar, garlic, soy sauce, and bay leaf over moderate heat.
2. Heat the mixture until it boils. Now, remove the mixture from the heat and put aside.

3. In a relatively large saucepan, heat the olive oil and add the yellow onion. Continue to fry the onion turns soft and lightly golden.

4. Add the chicken stock and make it boil before adding the soy sauce mixture, chicken, and couscous.

5. Continue boiling for about 5 minutes before reducing the heat.

6. Add the bok choy and boil again until the bok choy is tender.

7. Get rid of the bay leaf.

8. Scoop into warmed individual bowls and garnish with the green onions.

9. Serve immediately while still hot.

Nutritional Information per Serving

Serving Amount: 2 cups

Calories	240	Total carbohydrate	28g
Saturated fat	1g	Dietary fiber	4g
Total fat	4g	Sodium	828mg
Trans fat	0g	Protein	23g
Monounsaturated fat	1g	Cholesterol	56mg
Added sugars	0g		

Quick bean and tuna salad

Number of servings: 4

Ingredients

- 1/2whole-grain baguette, torn into 2-inch pieces
- 3tablespoons olive oil
- One 16-ounce can cannellini beans, drained and rinsed
- 2small dill pickles, cut into bite-sized pieces
- 1small red onion, thinly sliced
- 1tablespoons red wine vinegar
- 1/4teaspoon pepper
- 7-ounce pouch tuna, no salt added, drained and rinsed
- 2tablespoons finely chopped fresh parsley

Instructions

1. Preheat the grill for a few minutes.
2. Place the baguette pieces on a heavy cookie sheet and brush with 1 tablespoon of the oil.
3. Position cookie sheet under heat for about 1 to 2 minutes, until the pieces turn golden.
4. Roll the bread pieces and roast them for an additional 1 or 2 minutes.
5. In a relatively large bowl, mix the pickles, onion, vinegar, beans, pepper, and the remaining oil.

6. Fold the broiled baguette pieces.
7. Divide the mixture onto four plates or bowls and coat using the tuna and parsley.
8. Serve immediately.

Nutritional Information per Serving

Serving Amount: About 1 and 1/3 cups

Calories	316	Dietary fiber	7g
Cholesterol	15mg	Sodium	505mg
Total fat	12g	Total carbohydrate	31g
Monounsaturated fat	7g	Added sugars	0g
Saturated fat	1.5g	Trans fat	0g
Protein	21g		

15 Snack Recipes

Broccoli and Cheese Mini Egg Omelets

Number of Servings: 2

Ingredients

- 4 cups broccoli florets
- 4whole eggs
- 1cup egg whites
- 1/4cup reduced fat cheddar
- 1/4 cup grated Romano or parmesan cheese
- 1tablespoon olive oil
- Salt and fresh pepper
- Cooking spray

Instructions:

1. Preheat oven to about 175 C.
2. In a medium-sized pan, steam broccoli with in some water for about 6-7 minutes.
3. After broccoli is completely cooked, crush into smaller pieces and add olive oil, salt and pepper, and mix well.
4. Sprinkle muffin tins with cooking spray and scoop the broccoli mixture evenly into 9 tins.
5. Beat eggs, grated parmesan cheese, salt, egg whites, and pepper in a medium bowl to form a mixture.

6. Scoop the mixture in the greased tins over broccoli until a bit more than half full.
7. Cover the ingredients with shredded cheddar
8. Bake in an oven for about 20 minutes.
9. Remove from the oven and serve immediately.

Note: You can wrap any leftovers in plastic wrap and store in the refrigerator to enjoy a few times in the course of the week.

Nutritional Information per Serving

Serving Amount: 2 serving spoons

Calories	84	Sodium	332mg
Total fat	6g	Total carbohydrate	7g
Saturated fat	2g	Dietary fiber	2g
Monounsaturated fat	10g	Total sugars	0g
Cholesterol	13mg	Protein	12g
Trans fat	9g		

Sweet and spicy snack mix

Number of Servings: 12

Ingredients

- 2 cans (15 ounces each) garbanzos (Rinsed, drained and patted dry)
- 2cups wheat squares cereal
- 1cup dried pineapple chunks
- 1cup raisins
- 2tablespoons honey
- 2tablespoons Worcestershire sauce
- 1teaspoon garlic powder
- 1/2 teaspoon chili powder

Instructions

1. Heat the oven to 175 C.
2. Sparingly spray 15 x 10 baking sheet with butter-flavored cooking spray and put it aside.
3. Spray a heavy skillet using the same butter-flavored cooking spray and add garbanzos. Cook over medium heat and ensure that you keep stirring frequently until the beans start to turn to brown.
4. Now, transfer the garbanzos to the ready baking sheet.

5. Continue to lightly spray the beans with cooking spray and bake while stirring frequently until the beans are brittle. This should be about 20 minutes.

6. Cover a roasting pan with the cooking spray.

7. Put the cereal, pineapple, and raisins into the pan and add the roasted garbanzos while stirring to mix uniformly.

8. Take a large bowl and mix the spices, honey, and Worcestershire sauce while stirring to mix evenly. Pour the mixture over the snack mix and whisk gently.

9. Spray the mixture again with the cooking spray and bake for additional 10 to 15 minutes and stir occasionally to keep the mixture from burning or sticking to the pan.

10. Remove the ingredients from the oven and let cool.

11. Store in an airtight container for more servings within the next 2 or 3 days. (in the upcoming snack times).

Nutritional Information per Serving

Serving Amount: 1/2cup

Calorie	194	Total carbohydrate	39g
Cholesterol	0mg	Protein	5g
Monounsaturated fat	0.5g	Dietary fiber	5g
Total fat2 g	2g	Added sugars	3g
Trans fat	0g	Sodium	218mg

Peanut butter hummus

Number of Servings: 10 - 15

Ingredients

- 2 cups garbanzo beans
- 1cup water
- 1/2 cup powdered peanut butter
- 1/4cup natural peanut butter
- 2tablespoons brown sugar
- 1teaspoon vanilla extract

Instructions

1. Put all of the ingredients in a blender or food processor.
2. Blend until the resulting fluid becomes smooth.
3. Serve and consume immediately.
4. Refrigerate the remaining portion for a period not exceeding 5 days.

Nutritional Information per Serving

Serving Amount: 1/2glass

Calories	135	Sodium	47mg
Cholesterol	0mg	Total carbohydrate	19g
Saturated fat	0g	Protein	7g
Monounsaturated fat	1g	Dietary fiber	4g
Total fat	4g	Total sugars	4g
Trans fat	0g		

Avocado deviled eggs

Number of Servings: 6

Ingredients

- 6 eggs, hard boiled
- 1ripe avocado, peeled and pitted
- 1 1/2 teaspoons lime juice
- 3tablespoons light mayonnaise
- 1teaspoon chopped parsley
- 2teaspoons ground cayenne pepper
- 2cloves fresh garlic, minced

Instructions

1. Cut all the eggs lengthwise and detach the yolks and set aside.
2. In a medium-sized bowl, combine the egg yolks, half of the parsley, cayenne pepper mayonnaise, avocado, lime juice, and garlic.
3. Scoop the mixture into egg whites and decorate with other half of chopped parsley.
4. Serve immediately.

Nutritional Information per Serving

Serving Amount: 2 half portions

Calories	97	Sodium	126mg
Total fat	7g	Dietary fiber	2g
Saturated fat	1.5g	Total carbohydrate	3.5g
Monounsaturated fat	4g	Added sugar	0g
Cholesterol	93mg	Protein	5g
Trans fat	0g		

Spinach dip with mushrooms

Number of Servings: 10

Ingredients

- 1package (10 ounces) frozen chopped spinach (thawed and squeezed dry)
- 1 ½ cups fat-free sour cream
- 1cup fat-free mayonnaise
- 1cup chopped fresh mushrooms
- 3 green onions, chopped

Instructions

1. Mix all the ingredients in a medium-sized bowl.
2. Blend well, cover, and put in a fridge for around 10-15 minutes.
3. Serve frozen with a variety of raw vegetables.

Nutritional Information per Serving

Serving Amount: 1/2cup

Calories	56	Protein	3g
Cholesterol	3mg	Sodium	268mg
Trans fat	0g	Total carbohydrate	11g

Dietary fiber   1g   Total sugars   2g
Added sugars   0g

Orange juice smoothie

Number of Servings: 2

Ingredients

- 1cup fat-free vanilla frozen yogurt
- 3/4cup fat-free milk
- 1/4 cup frozen orange juice concentrate

Instructions

1. In a blender, mix all the ingredients.
2. Blend for around 10 minutes until the mixture becomes smooth.
3. Pour into a glass and serve immediately.
4. Refrigerate the surplus mixture up to 3 days

Nutritional Information per Serving

Serving Amount: 1 cup

Calories	180	Sodium	33mg
Cholesterol	2mg	Total carbohydrate	38g
Saturated fat	0g	Dietary fiber	0.5g
Protein	7g	Added sugars	22g
Trans fat	0g		

Lemon cheesecake

Number of Servings: 8

Ingredients

- 2tablespoons cold water
- 1envelope unflavored gelatin
- 2tablespoons lemon juice
- 1/2cup skim milk, heated almost to boiling
- Egg substitute equivalent to 1 or 2 egg whites
- 1/4cup sugar
- 1teaspoon vanilla
- 2cups low-fat cottage cheese
- Lemon zest

Instructions

1. Mix water, gelatin, and lemon juice in a blender and blend on slow speed for 3 minutes.
2. Add hot milk and continue blending until all gelatin is dissolved.
3. Into the resulting mixture, add egg substitute, vanilla, cheese, and sugar and process on high speed until smooth.
4. Pour into round flat dish and refrigerate up to 3 hours.
5. Coat using grated lemon zest before serving.

Nutritional Information per Serving

Serving Amount: 1/8 of cake

Calories	80	Sodium	252mg
Cholesterol	3mg	Total carbohydrate	9g
Total fat	1g	Protein	9g
Trans fat	0g	Added sugars	9g

Fresh fruit kebabs

Number of Servings: 2

Ingredients

- 6 ounces low-fat, sugar-free lemon yogurt
- 1 teaspoon fresh lime juice
- 1 teaspoon lime zest
- 4 pineapple chunks (about 1/2-inch each)
- 4 strawberries
- 1 kiwi, peeled and quartered
- 1/2 banana, cut into four 1/2 -inch chunks
- 4 red grapes
- Four wooden skewers

Instructions

1. In a relatively small bowl, beat together the lime zest, lime juice, and yogurt.
2. Cover with foil and refrigerate for about 30 minutes.
3. Slice 1 of each fruit onto each of the skewers.
4. Now retrieve the refrigerated mixture and serve in a glass together with the lemon lime dip.

Nutritional Information per Serving

Serving Amount: 2 fruit kebabs

Calories	190	Sodium	52mg
Cholesterol	5mg	Total carbohydrate	39mg
Added sugars	6g	Dietary fiber	4g
Total fat	2g	Saturated fat	1g
Trans fat	0g	Protein	4g

Cookies and cream shake

Number of Servings: 3

Ingredients

- 1 ½ cups vanilla soy milk (soya milk), chilled
- 3 cups fat-free vanilla ice cream
- 6chocolate wafer cookies, crushed

Instructions

1. In a blender, mix soy milk and ice cream and blend until frothy and smooth.
2. Add cookies and blend again.
3. Pour into a glass and serve immediately.

Nutritional Information per Serving

Serving Amount: 1 cup (generous)

Calories	270	Total carbohydrate	52g
Monounsaturated fat	Less than 1g	Dietary fiber	11.5g
Saturated fat	Less than 1g	Total fat	3g

Trans fat	0g	Sodium	224mg
Protein	9g	Total sugars	29g
Added sugars	11g		

Whole-wheat pretzel

Number of Servings: 12

Ingredients

- 1package active dry yeast
- 2teaspoon brown sugar
- 1/2teaspoon kosher salt
- 1 ½ cups warm water
- 1 cup bread flour
- 3cups whole-wheat flour
- 1 tablespoon olive oil
- 1/2cup wheat gluten
- Cooking spray
- 1/4cup baking soda
- 1egg white or 1/4cup egg-substitute

Instructions

1. In the bowl of a food processor, dissolve sugar, salt, and yeast into warm water and set aside for around 5 minutes.
2. Add olive oil, gluten, and flours and mix by hand for about 5 minutes until a smooth dough forms.
3. Spray inside of bowl surface with cooking spray to avoid dough from sticking.
4. Cover the dough using a plastic lid and place in warm place for about 1 hour or until doubled in size.

5. Strike the dough down and divide into 12 pieces before rolling into long ropes.

6. Make U-shape with a single rope, one at a time, and then cross ends over and pinch in the bottom of the U-shape. This can be deemed to be the same as making the traditional pretzel shape.

7. To about 8 cups of boiling water, add 1/4cup baking soda and pretzels (one at a time) and cook for about 1 minute.

8. Remove the pretzels using a cooking stick or spatula to parchment-lined baking pan.

9. Brush with egg white or egg-substitute and bake for 15 minutes in a 235 C.

10. Cool and serve immediately

Nutritional Information per Serving

Serving Amount: 1 pretzel

Calorie	182	Dietary fiber	4g
Monounsaturated fat	1g	Total carbohydrate	31g
Trans fat	0g	Sodium	108mg
Total fat	2g	Protein	10g
Added sugars	1g		

Morning glory muffins

Number of Servings: 15 - 18

Ingredients

- 1cup all-purpose (plain) flour
- 1cup whole-wheat flour
- 3/4cup sugar
- 2 teaspoons baking soda
- 2 teaspoons ground cinnamon
- 3/4 cup egg substitute
- 1/2 cup vegetable oil
- 1/2 cup unsweetened applesauce
- 2 teaspoons vanilla extract
- 2 cups chopped apples (unpeeled)
- 1/2 cup raisins
- 3/4 cup grated carrots
- 2tablespoons chopped pecans

Instructions

1. Heat the oven to 175 C.
2. Cover a muffin pan with foil lining.
3. Mix the sugar, baking soda, flours, and cinnamon in a relatively large bowl and beat to blend evenly.
4. Mix the egg substitute, oil, applesauce, and vanilla in a separate bowl. Stir in the raisins, carrots, and apple.

5. Add to the flour mixture and blend until it becomes moistened and slightly lumpy.
6. Scoop the batter into muffin cups fill each to about 2/3 full.
7. Coat with chopped pecans and bake for about 35 minutes until bouncy to the touch.
8. Set aside to completely cool for 15-20 minutes.
9. Serve with your favorite beverage.

Nutritional Information per Serving

Serving Amount: 1 muffin

Calories	175	Sodium	163mg
Total fat	7g	Total carbohydrate	25g
Saturated fat	0.5g	Dietary fiber	2g
Monounsaturated fat	4g	Total sugars	13g
Protein	3g	Added sugars	8g

Muesli breakfast bars

Number of Servings: 8 - 12

Ingredients

- Two 1/2 cups old-fashioned rolled oats
- 1/2 cup soy flour
- 1/2 cup fat-free dry milk
- 1/2 cup toasted wheat germ
- 1/2cup sliced (flaked) almonds or chopped pecans, toasted
- 1/2cup dried apples, chopped
- 1/2 cup raisins
- 1/2 teaspoon salt
- 1cup dark honey
- 1/2cup natural unsalted peanut butter
- 1tablespoon olive oil
- 2teaspoons vanilla extract

Instructions

1. Preheat the oven to 165 C.
2. Sparingly coat a 13 x 9-inch baking pan using olive oil cooking spray.
3. In a relatively large bowl, mix the dry milk, wheat germ, almonds, oats, apples, raisins, salt, and flour. Whip well to blend and put aside until needed.

4. In a saucepan, mix the honey, peanut butter, and olive oil under low heat until completely blended.

5. Before the mixture comes to boil, add in the vanilla while stirring.

6. Now, add the warm honey mixture to the dry ingredients and stir quickly until everything blends completely. Ensure that the mixture is sticky but not wet.

7. Pat the mixture uniformly into a ready baking pan and press firmly to get rid of any air pockets.

8. Bake until the edges start to turn golden brown for about 25 minutes.

9. Withdraw it from the heat to allow cooling for about 10 minutes before cutting into 24 bars.

10. When the bars are cool and can be handled with bare hands, remove them from the pan and serve immediately.

11. Refrigerate the surplus bars in an airtight container.

Nutritional Information per Serving

Serving Amount: 2 bars

Calories	177	Sodium	75mg
Total carbohydrate	27g	Dietary fiber	3g
Saturated fat	1g	Cholesterol	1mg
Total fat	5g	Protein	6g
Trans fat	0g	Monounsaturated fat	2g
Added sugars	11g		

Mushroom barley soup

Number of Servings: 9

Ingredients

- 1 tablespoon canola oil
- 1 ½ cups chopped onions
- 1 cup sliced mushrooms
- 3/4 cup chopped carrots
- 1 teaspoon dried thyme
- 1/8 teaspoon black pepper
- 1/2 teaspoon chopped garlic
- 8 cups vegetable stock
- 3/4 cup pearl barley
- 3 ounces dry sherry
- 1/2 small potato, chopped
- 1/4 cup thinly sliced green onions

Instructions

1. Heat the canola oil in a large stock pot under medium heat.
2. Add the thyme, pepper, onions, carrots, garlic, and mushrooms and fry until the onion turns translucent. This should be for about 5 minutes.
3. Add the vegetable stock and barley and boil with high heat for about 5 minutes.

4. Lessen the heat and simmer until barley is tender for about 15 minutes

5. Add and stir the sherry and potato and continue to simmer until the potato is cooked, about 15 minutes.

6. Decorate with sliced green onions before serving.

Nutritional Information per Serving

Serving Amount: 8 ounces

Calories	121	Sodium	112mg
Cholesterol	0mg	Total carbohydrate	19g
Saturated fat	0g	Dietary fiber	3g
Total fat	4g	Total sugars	2g
Monounsaturated fat	3g	Protein	2g
Trans fat	0g		

Pizza Margherita

Number of Servings: 6

Ingredients

Whole-grain pizza dough:

- 1 teaspoon active dry yeast
- 3/4 cup warm water
- 3/4 cup whole-wheat flour
- 2 tablespoons barley flour
- 2 teaspoons gluten
- 1 tablespoon oats
- 1 tablespoon olive oil

Toppings:

- Two 1/2 cups chopped spinach
- Two 1/2 cups sliced tomatoes
- 1/4 cup chopped basil
- 1 tablespoon minced oregano
- 1 tablespoon minced garlic
- 1 teaspoon black pepper
- 2 ounces of fresh mozzarella

Instructions

1. Add water in a large bowl and slowly add both whole wheat and barley flour and make dough. Set it aside for about 5 minutes.
2. Dissolve yeast in warm water.
3. Combine the dry ingredients in a medium-sized bowl and then add oil and the water-yeast mixture.
4. Press with a spatula for 10-15 minutes to attain a smooth texture.
5. Refrigerate the dough and let it rise for a minimum of 1 hour.
6. Heat oven to 230 C.
7. Make dough balls and compress them on a floured surface to 1/4-inch thickness.
8. Put the dough on baking sheet and coat with tomatoes, basil, garlic, black pepper, spinach, mozzarella, and oregano.
9. Bake until all the cheese melts and the crust is crispy. This should be within 10-15 minutes.
10. Withdraw from the oven and let cool for about 10 minutes before serving.

Nutritional Information per Serving

Serving Amount: 1 slice of pizza

| Calories | 144 | Sodium | 83mg |
| Cholesterol | 6mg | Total carbohydrate | 20g |

Saturated fat	1g	Dietary fiber	6g
Total fat	5g	Trans fat	0g
Protein	7g	Monounsaturated fat	2g
Added sugars	0g		

Shrimp Ceviche

Number of servings: 5 - 8

Ingredients

- 1/2-pound raw shrimp, cut in Quarter inch pieces
- 2 lemons, zest and juice
- 2 limes, zest and juice
- 2 tablespoons olive oil
- 2 teaspoons cumin
- 1/2cup diced red onion
- 1cup diced tomato
- 2tablespoons minced garlic
- 1cup black beans, cooked
- 1/4cup diced serrano chili pepper and seeds removed
- 1cup diced cucumber, peeled and seeded
- 1/4 cup chopped cilantro

Instructions

1. Put shrimp in a relatively shallow pan and mix with lemon and lime juices and reserve the rest.
2. Freezeuntil shrimp is rigid and white for at least 3 hours.
3. While shrimp is freezing, combine the remaining ingredients in a separate bowl and set aside.
4. Mix shrimp and citrus juice with remaining ingredients.

5. Serve immediately with baked tortilla chips.

Nutritional Information per Serving

Serving Amount: About 3/4cup

Calories	100	Sodium	168mg
Saturated fat	2g	Total carbohydrate	12g
Cholesterol	34mg	Dietary fiber	4g
Monounsaturated fat	3g	Added sugars	0g
Total fat	4g	Protein	8g

Chapter Six

Additional Information

About The Dash Diet

FAQs about the DASH Diet

Can I still go on the DASH diet even if I don't have high blood pressure?

Of course! Originally, the DASH diet was designed for patients with high blood pressure. Nonetheless, it is focused on healthy foods that make it suitable for anyone, regardless of having high blood pressure or not.

For how long should I stay on the DASH diet?

Nutritionists get this question a lot. However, the answer is simple! The DASH diet is intended to be a life-long change in your eating habits. It positively impacts on your cooking and eating skills and even allows you to occasionally overindulge.

How long will it take before I see the results?

With the proper and efficient use of the diet, you can get results by the end of the second week. The DASH diet is proven to have both short- and long-term impact on weight loss. You can lose even more pounds if you effectively utilize the DASH diet.

What should I drink while on the DASH diet?

It is evident that you may prefer a certain drink; water is the best option while on this diet. Naturally, water is the best hydrating solution and doesn't have calories, added sugars, or sodium.

Can a vegetarian cope well with the DASH diet?

Whilst the DASH diet integrates the eating of six or fewer pieces of lean meat, you do not have to consume it! For a vegetarian, you can substitute meat with beans, chickpeas, or any other type of cereals that have a high level of protein.

Why does the DASH diet strongly limit the intake of sodium?

High intake of large amounts of foods that are deemed to contain large volumes of sodium can play a role in heightening blood pressure. The DASH diet was primarily createdto control this menace. Therefore, the plan advocates for the reduction of sodium consumption.

Can I consume caffeine or alcohol while on the diet?

Surprisingly, the DASH diet doesn't deny you the pleasure you derive from either caffeine or alcohol. However, the diet plan recommends some limits which should be adhered to. If you have to drink them, try having only caffeine with meals and don't have more than two cans of alcoholic beverages.

While taking specific medications, could this diet change how they work?

It is always prudent to take the advice of your doctor about consumption of foods while on specific medications. Certain medication needs you to have various varieties of foods. While taking any type of medication, note that the DASH diet should be taken with a prior consultation with a doctor.

What if I do not witness any changes within the first month while doing the DASH diet?

Once you feel as if the DASH diet has had no impact on your condition, do not jump to the conclusion that it doesn't work. Rather, visit your doctor and get a screening. You probably could have other medical problems that are inhibiting the efficiency of the DASH diet. Mind you, the DASH diet has been proven to work for the last few decades.

If you happen to have any other questions about the DASH diet, feel free to visit any Registered Dietitian Nutritionist (RDN) or doctor for more advice.

The Pros and Cons of the DASH Diet Plan

Just like any other medicine, nutritional advice, or regimen to improve health, the DASH diet plan has a few pros and cons as discussed below.

Pros

There are no special foods required since the DASH diet plan comprises a variety of foods that are readily available. The only goal is to eat a certain serving size of each food category. The food items and ingredients integrated into this plan can easily be found at any grocery store at an affordable price.

The DASH diet plan is readily cost-effective, accessible, and affordable on online platforms. Moreover, there are nutritionists who can give you a copy of the plan after a consultation.

The plan is very flexible and is designed to have a variety of calorie levels that one can choose from. The most effective calorie level to be utilized can be in line with the advice of a nutritionist. In most cases, the calorie level selected is based on body weight as well as the intensity of hypertension in an individual. Since a desire for weight loss may be a long-term strategy, one can use the appropriate calorie levels in a progressive way for maximum impact.

Immense improvement of health has been witnessed and the DASH diet is proven to be effective in reducing blood pressure and cholesterol. Nonetheless, the health benefits are greatly evident when the plan is consistently adhered to.

There are humongous nutritional benefits that emanate from using the DASH diet plan. For this reason, the DASH diet plan has been supported by various nutritionists and major health organizations.

Unlike other types of diet plans, the DASH diet allows one to enjoy other types of food and instead gives a limit which should be adhered to.

Cons

There is no restaurant that is known to always have a prepared DASH diet meal. This means that one has to always go the freezer section at the nearest grocery shop and purchase the ingredients. To some, this is somehow inconvenient.

Whilst many people may be using the DASH diet plan solely to reduce weight, the plan is partially designed for this purpose. The primary emphasis of this plan is to work on your hypertensive condition.

The plan is against the use of high levels of sodium intake. However, we cannot fail to notice that the sodium minerals are very important in a number of bodily processes.

Thank You!

Before you go, I would like to thank you for purchasing a copy of our book. Out of the dozens of books you could have picked, you decided to go with this one and for that I are very grateful.

I hope you enjoyed reading it as much as I enjoyed writing it! I hope you found it very informative.

I would like to ask you for a small favor. <u>Could you please take a moment to leave a review for this book on Amazon?</u>

Your feedback will help me continue to write more books and release new content in the future!